Strengthen Your Mind Volume Two

Strengthen Your Mind Volume Two
Activities for People Concerned About Early Memory Loss

by

Kristin Einberger

and

Janelle Sellick

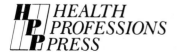
HEALTH
PROFESSIONS
PRESS

Baltimore • London • Sydney

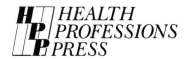

Health Professions Press, Inc.
Post Office Box 10624
Baltimore, Maryland 21285-0624

www.healthpropress.com

Typeset by Barton Matheson Willse & Worthington, Baltimore, Maryland.
Manufactured in the United States of America by Versa Press, East Peoria, Illinois.

The following title is also available from Health Professions Press, Inc.:

Strengthen Your Mind, Volume One

To order, contact Health Professions Press, Inc., Post Office Box 10624, Baltimore, MD 21285-0624 (1-888-337-8808); http://www.healthpropress.com

Library of Congress Cataloging-in-Publication Data

Einberger, Kristin.
  Strengthen your mind, volume two : activities for people concerned about early memory loss / by Kristin Einberger and Janelle Sellick.
    p.   cm.
  ISBN-13: 978-1-932529-42-5
  1. Memory disorders—Exercise therapy.   I. Sellick, Janelle.   II. Title.
  BF376.E36 2007
  616.8'3—dc22   2006029586

British Library Cataloguing in Publication data are available from the British Library.

Contents

Preface vii

Acknowledgments ix

Introduction 1

People 5

    Athletes of Greatness 7

    The A–Z of Famous People from the United States 9

    The Brides and Grooms 11

    The Creative Spirit 13

    Distinguished Women 15

    Expressions Related to People 19

    Famous Scandals 21

    Famous Child Actors 23

    Famous Couples 25

    Famous "Doubles" 27

    Famous People and the Occupations that Made Them So 29

    Famous People Defined by Their Hairstyles and Hats 31

    Famous Siblings 33

    First Ladies 35

    Leaders in the World of Science and Nature 37

    Military Leaders 39

    People and Characters Who Come in Threes 41

    People Known by Initials in Their Name 43

    People with Food Products Named After Them 45

    Places and Things Named for People 47

    Popular Song Titles that Contain a Person's Name 49

    Presidential Facts 51

    Terms for Groups of People 53

    Time Magazine Person of the Year 55

    Television Hosts 57

    Who Invented What? 59

    Who Wrote What? 61

    The World of Music 63

Places 65

    At the Baseball Park and on the Golf Course 67

    At the Movies 69

    The A–Z of U.S. Cities 71

    Early Homes of U.S. Presidents 73

    The East Coast 75

    The High Seas 77

    Home Sweet Home 79

    In the Neighborhood 81

    In the Universe 83

    Legendary Places 85

    Main Street, USA 87

    Nicknames and Historical Names of Countries around the World 89

On the Map 91
On the Road 93
Out in the Cold. 95
People and Places. 97
Places Animals Live 99
Places Associated with the Seasons. 101
Places that Are Also Things 103
Settings of Famous Events 105
Some Like It Hot. 107
Songs with Geographical Names in the Titles. 109
Space and Beyond 113
This Is the Place 115
The West Coast 117
Which Continent Is It?. 119
Which Country Is It? 121
Which State Is It? 123

Things. 129
All About Arches 131
All-American Things 133
Animal Facts 135
Animal Sayings. 137
The Color of Money. 139
Comedy, Laughter, and Smiles. 141
Events that Changed History 143
Expressions with Body Parts 145
Expressions with Colors 147
Expressions with Foods. 149
Expressions with Numbers. 151
Fabulous in Fives 153
Famous Brand-Names. 155
Famous Recipes 157
Food around the United States 159
Important Dates in History. 161
In the Dark. 163
In the Middle of Things. 165
Man's Best Friend. 167
Mothers and Fathers 169
Over and Under 171
Pass the Cheese, Please! 173
Passing Fads 175
Products with Numbers 177
Shoes. 179
Show Me the Money 181
The Sound of Music. 183
Things that Are Square 185
Things with a Letter in Their Name 187
What's What in American Business?. 189
Where on the Human Body? 191

Preface

The importance of taking part in mentally stimulating activities is becoming more apparent every day. Healthy older adults, people concerned about their memory, and individuals diagnosed with an early memory loss disorder can all benefit from keeping their minds active. As in Volume One of *Strengthen Your Mind*, the all-new worksheets in Volume Two are a wonderful resource to use in your quest to enhance memory and to sharpen your mind. Although completing the worksheets individually is an excellent way to challenge your mind, for an added bonus try completing them with a friend or family member. Adding this social component makes for even broader mental stimulation (and is fun, too!).

We have been thrilled with the interest shown in *Strengthen Your Mind, Volume One,* and continue to advocate for services for people with early memory loss. Through weekly early memory loss groups and presentations at various conferences throughout the United States, we have witnessed firsthand the need for resources designed specifically for people with early memory loss and those interested in enhancing their memory. As in Volume One, the worksheets in Volume Two have been field-tested with individuals in our early memory loss groups to ensure that the topics are interesting and that the level of difficulty is appropriate.

The groups with which we work continue to be our best teachers in designing and creating the content of the book. It is with much gratitude that we thank them!

Strengthen Your Mind, Volume One, is used by individuals and groups throughout the United States, and we are happy to report that we have received positive feedback about the usefulness of the manual. We hope that Volume Two will be equally useful as well as a welcome addition to *your* library!

Strengthen Your Mind, Volume Two, is dedicated to a group very near and dear to our hearts—Brain Boosters, an early memory loss program in Northern California. Since 2004, they have been our inspiration in the development and creation of activities specifically designed to focus on the strengths of this very hard-working and dedicated group of people.

Brain Boosters participants have "field-tested" many of the activities contained within this book and have made helpful suggestions that have resulted in positive changes to our writing each step of the way. They are an invaluable resource for people throughout the United States who are dealing with early memory loss. To them we offer our heartfelt gratitude for their advice and our everlasting appreciation for exemplifying the dedication of the millions of people throughout the world who are working diligently to enhance their memory.

Acknowledgments

From Kristin: To my sons Derek and Scott, your love and support throughout have had a great impact on my being able to actually finish this book! To my mom, Elenka, your ideas and everlasting support have been invaluable. You're the greatest! And to Anne, thanks so much for listening, for lending support, for offering advice and ideas, and for editing over and over again. You are all at the top of my list!!!

From Janelle: To my husband Mike, thank you for all of your ideas and suggestions and for encouraging me along the way—your support means so much to me. To my girls, Megan, Mia, and Josie, thank you for putting up with all of my hours in front of the computer—Mommy loves you! And to my mom and dad, thank you for your ideas and interest in my work—I appreciate all of your help!

Introduction

For years it was thought that there was little that could be done to strengthen the minds of those with memory loss. Today, thanks to the dedication of many, we know differently. Listening to or playing music, exercising, eating foods high in antioxidants, socializing, learning new things, doing things differently, doing crossword puzzles and other cognitively stimulating activities—all of these are becoming more and more prevalent as ways to enhance a person's memory.

Since our first book, *Strengthen Your Mind: Activities for People with Early Memory Loss, Volume One,* was written, mental stimulation as a means to strengthen memory has gained a great deal of attention. It is hard to pick up a magazine or newspaper without seeing some mention of this fact. Although a cure for Alzheimer's disease and other forms of dementia has not yet become a reality, research is identifying many exciting new discoveries that can make positive differences in the lives of those who are dealing with early memory loss.

The 87 all-new activities (or worksheets) within this manual are designed to make a positive difference by enhancing memory as well as by creating an outlet for socialization, pure enjoyment, and fun. The worksheets will encourage you to research and discuss a variety of topics that you may never have had an interest in or even thought of learning about before. With each worksheet that you complete, you will gain a little more knowledge to tuck away and add to a lifetime of learning and experiences. Do not worry if you cannot find the answer to every question; just enjoy taking the time to find the answers by talking with others or using reference materials such as the Internet, dictionaries, and encyclopedias. You may find more than one answer for some questions. Above all, have fun using this manual—the true benefit of the worksheets is participating in the process of finding the answers, not knowing every answer!

In this second volume of *Strengthen Your Mind*, activities are divided into three sections—People, Places, and Things. The worksheets are in the same format as in Volume One. For each topic, on the front page is a short introduction and on the back page is an answer sheet. Answers are in a variety of forms, including multiple choice, fill in the blank, and brainstorming. Some answers will come easily. Others may necessitate some research. Using a map or globe will be helpful in working on activities that involve geography. Other worksheets, such as *Pass the Cheese, Please,* may call for a walk around the grocery store. And still others, such as *Important Dates in History,* may call for the use of an encyclopedia, the Internet, or a discussion with a history buff.

Our intent is that you use these worksheets as a means to enhance your memory, whether you know all of the answers or whether you need to do some research to find them. Remember, knowing the answers is not the important part of using this manual; using the worksheets to strengthen your mind and to provide enjoyment is! We wish you luck in your journey. You are to be commended for being proactive in dealing with your memory loss. Give yourself a pat on the back. Then wait no longer—get started on the activities!

INFORMATION FOR FACILITATORS

As with Volume One of *Strengthen Your Mind,* these worksheets are not only beneficial for individuals with early memory loss, but also for professionals (i.e., *facilitators*) who work with people who want to strengthen their minds. At the bottom of each *answer sheet,* below the answers to the questions, are suggestions for facilitators on ways to encourage further discussion on each topic. The worksheets are designed to be reproducible. We suggest making enough copies (front side only) for each person in your group. You may also want to provide extra copies for people to take home with them so that they can work together on a topic with family members or friends. Make sure that participants are relaxed and focused on the topic before starting to work on an activity. When reviewing the questions, encourage people in the group to share their answers. Avoid just "reading off" the answers, and take time to let people share any thoughts, memories, or stories that arise. Make the group feel comfortable by encouraging them to share or by sharing a story of your own. You can ask them how they liked the worksheet, if they found it easy or difficult, or with whom they worked to complete it.

We suggest that you use a map for any worksheet that involves geography. For those that involve food, taste tests would be fun. For those that involve music, try bringing in different types of music and instruments and encourage singing. An A–Z list of a topic within an activity may be a good spin-off exercise for many of the worksheets. Simply coming up with a list of things—such as things that fly when completing the *Space and Beyond* worksheet or a list of presidents of the United States when completing the *Presidential Facts* worksheet, would be a good exercise. For other worksheets, such as *Which State Is It?*, it may be a great time to do a sort of show and tell for which participants bring in pictures or items from states in which they were born or have lived. Using a variety of visual and auditory aids can be beneficial in working with all of the activities.

The most important aspect of these worksheets is their ability to serve as a means to reminisce, to learn new things, and to experience a sense of joy. We hope you and those with whom you work will find this manual to be a valuable tool and that it will have a positive impact on the lives of many.

People

Throughout history people and their beliefs have helped to shape the world. Major historical events and the people involved in them have been studied by scholars and lay people alike. The dictionary defines the word *people* as "human beings in general" or "the common persons of a nation." In this section there are 30 worksheets dedicated to people of all types. For example, you will find worksheets on historical figures, such as *Military Leaders*, as well as lighthearted worksheets, such as *Famous People Defined by Their Hairstyles and Hats*. Enjoy this section, and do not be afraid to ask other people to help you if you get stuck. After all, interacting with others is one of the best things that you can do to keep your mind sharp. So pick up the phone and call a friend or family member if you need some help!

Athletes of Greatness

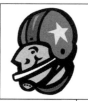

From the ancient Olympics, which began in 776 BC, to the modern Olympic games, which began in 1896, people have shown a great interest in watching sports and have revered great athletes. The truly great athletes often become "household names," even for those who are not particularly interested in the sport. Below are some facts regarding some of the most famous athletes of the last 100 years. Can you name them?

1. In 1926, this American female swimmer became the first woman to swim across the English Channel. Upon returning home, she received a very large ticker-tape parade in New York City.

2. This man, nicknamed "The Greatest," "the Champ," and "Louisville Lip," was one of the best heavyweight boxers of all time. He changed his birth name when he was a young man after he converted to Islam.

3. This runner won gold medals in both the decathlon and the pentathlon. He also excelled in many other sports, including football, baseball, and basketball. Being of mixed Native American and white ancestry, he struggled with racism throughout his sports career.

4. This great swimmer won an unprecedented seven events-all that he entered-in the 1972 summer Olympics in Germany. This record has yet to be broken.

5. Perhaps the most famous baseball player of all time, this New York Yankee "Sultan of Swat" held the home run record of 60 in a season, until Roger Maris broke it in the early 1960s. He changed the game of baseball with his power and his personality.

6. In 1947, this Brooklyn Dodger great became the first black major league baseball player in modern times. Inducted into the Hall of Fame in 1962, he was a member of six World Series winning teams and also won many other awards.

7. This man, one of the greatest golfers of all time, was nicknamed "The King." He won seven major championships between 1958 and 1964 and continued to play professionally until 2004.

8. This 7'1" basketball player was nicknamed " . . . the Stilt." He is the only player to average more than 50 points per game in a season and also the only one to score a whopping 100 points in a single game!

9. This female swimmer wrote an autobiography named *The Million Dollar Mermaid*. She went on from swimming to become a very successful movie star of the 1940s and '50s.

10. This world famous bike rider won an unprecedented seven consecutive Tour de France road races from 1999 to 2005. After courageously beating cancer, he began a foundation to fight the disease. His yellow "Live Strong" rubber bracelets have become popular throughout the world and have raised many millions of dollars to support his foundation.

11. This child prodigy began playing golf at age 2 and by age 8 was winning tournaments. In 2006, he was the highest paid athlete, winning $100 million in tournaments and endorsements! He has been the PGA Player of the Year eight times.

12. This football great spent most of his years as quarterback for the New York Jets, beginning in 1965. His antics, both on and off the field, were legendary. He appeared in many advertisements and was especially known for Remington electric shaver ads. His nickname is "Broadway . . . "

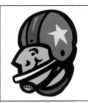

1. In 1926, this American female swimmer became the first woman to swim across the English Channel. Upon returning home, she received a very large ticker-tape parade in New York City.
   Gertrude Ederle

2. This man, nicknamed "The Greatest," "the Champ," and "Louisville Lip," was one of the best heavyweight boxers of all time. He changed his birth name when he was a young man after he converted to Islam.
   Mohammed Ali

3. This runner won gold medals in both the decathlon and the pentathlon. He also excelled in many other sports, including football, baseball, and basketball. Being of mixed Native American and white ancestry, he struggled with racism throughout his sports career.
   Jim Thorpe

4. This great swimmer won an unprecedented seven events-all that he entered-in the 1972 summer Olympics in Germany. This record has yet to be broken.
   Mark Spitz

5. Perhaps the most famous baseball player of all time, this New York Yankee "Sultan of Swat" held the home run record of 60 in a season, until Roger Maris broke it in the early 1960s. He changed the game of baseball with his power and his personality.
   Babe Ruth

6. In 1947, this Brooklyn Dodger great became the first black major league baseball player in modern times. Inducted into the Hall of Fame in 1962, he was a member of six World Series winning teams and also won many other awards.
   Jackie Robinson

7. This man, one of the greatest golfers of all time, was nicknamed "The King." He won seven major championships between 1958 and 1964 and continued to play professionally until 2004.
   Arnold Palmer

8. This 7'1" basketball player was nicknamed " . . . the Stilt." He is the only player to average more than 50 points per game in a season and also the only one to score a whopping 100 points in a single game!
   Wilt Chamberlin

9. This female swimmer wrote an autobiography named *The Million Dollar Mermaid*. She went on from swimming to become a very successful movie star of the 1940s and '50s.
   Esther Williams

10. This world famous bike rider won an unprecedented seven consecutive Tour de France road races from 1999 to 2005. After courageously beating cancer, he began a foundation to fight the disease. His yellow "Live Strong" rubber bracelets have become popular throughout the world and have raised many millions of dollars to support his foundation.
    Lance Armstrong

11. This child prodigy began playing golf at age 2 and by age 8 was winning tournaments. In 2006, he was the highest paid athlete, winning $100 million in tournaments and endorsements! He has been the PGA Player of the Year eight times.
    Tiger Woods

12. This football great spent most of his years as quarterback for the New York Jets, beginning in 1965. His antics, both on and off the field, were legendary. He appeared in many advertisements and was especially known for Remington electric shaver ads. His nickname is "Broadway . . ."
    Joe Namath

FACILITATOR: These athletes represent a number of different sports. Do participants think that these people are the best in their field? Who do they think are the greatest athletes of all time? Which sports do participants like best? Would they rather watch or participate? Which sports did they play in school? It would be beneficial to have pictures of these athletes, if possible. You might also want to bring in equipment from some different sports and ask participants to identify the sport and a "great" that might have used the equipment.

The A–Z of Famous People from the United States

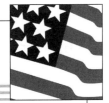

How many famous people from the United States can you name for each letter of the alphabet? You may use either first or last name. Famous people may include those from history, inventions, science, sports, music, television, movies, and more.

A

B

C

D

E

F

G

H

I

J

K

L

M

N

O

P

Q

R

S

T

U

V

W

X

Y

Z

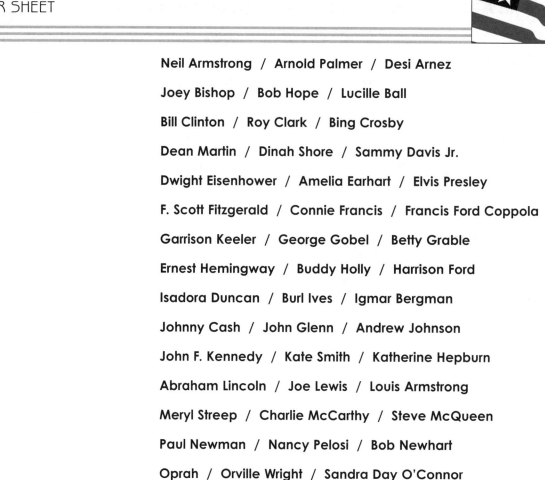

A	Neil Armstrong / Arnold Palmer / Desi Arnez
B	Joey Bishop / Bob Hope / Lucille Ball
C	Bill Clinton / Roy Clark / Bing Crosby
D	Dean Martin / Dinah Shore / Sammy Davis Jr.
E	Dwight Eisenhower / Amelia Earhart / Elvis Presley
F	F. Scott Fitzgerald / Connie Francis / Francis Ford Coppola
G	Garrison Keeler / George Gobel / Betty Grable
H	Ernest Hemingway / Buddy Holly / Harrison Ford
I	Isadora Duncan / Burl Ives / Igmar Bergman
J	Johnny Cash / John Glenn / Andrew Johnson
K	John F. Kennedy / Kate Smith / Katherine Hepburn
L	Abraham Lincoln / Joe Lewis / Louis Armstrong
M	Meryl Streep / Charlie McCarthy / Steve McQueen
N	Paul Newman / Nancy Pelosi / Bob Newhart
O	Oprah / Orville Wright / Sandra Day O'Connor
P	George Patton / Sidney Poitier / Perry Como
Q	Quincy Jones / Queen Latifah / John Quincy Adams
R	Babe Ruth / Rosemary Clooney / Paul Revere
S	John Steinbeck / Barbra Streisand / Frank Sinatra
T	Ty Cobb / Thomas Edison / Elizabeth Taylor
U	Ulysses S. Grant / Johnny Unitas / Ursula Andress
V	Vic Damone / Victor Borge / Vivian Vance
W	Tiger Woods / Wyatt Earp / Will Rogers
X	I couldn't find any. Can you?
Y	Glenn Yarborough / Brigham Young / Yul Brenner
Z	Zachary Taylor / Zsa Zsa Gabor / Zane Gray

FACILITATOR: *Above are examples that can be given when participants get stuck. You can also give clues to elicit the above examples once others are discussed. You can use this A–Z format for an endless assortment of activities. Try an A–Z list of cars, fruits and vegetables, candy bars, countries, businesses, and more.*

The Bride and Groom

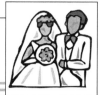

The first civilization to recognize marriage in law was Ancient Egypt. Much has changed since those times thousands of years ago, but the institution of marriage still remains. It is celebrated in a variety of ways in different parts of the world, and is more often a celebration of the joining in matrimony of a couple. The following activity is based on brides, grooms, and marriages.

1. The future groom is the special guest at this party, usually held a day or two before the wedding.

2. These judges, though not religious officials, often perform civil marriage ceremonies.

3. The white wedding gown is a tradition begun by this 19th-century Queen of England.

4. This city in Nevada is the setting for thousands of civil wedding ceremonies each year.

5. Finish this common saying referring to what the bride-to-be should wear: "Something old, something new, . . ."

6. This is another word for trousseau, the gifts that a bride's family typically gives to the family of the groom.

7. This is what many grooms do as the married couple enters their home for the first time.

8. In many Asian countries, the wedding gown is this color, a "happy" color.

9. The main member of the bride's wedding party is named this.

10. If an unmarried woman catches this, it is said that she will be the next to be married.

11. If an unmarried man catches this, he, too, will be the next to be married!

12. A legal contract entered into by the couple prior to the wedding is called a what?

13. CNN/Money found that the average cost of a wedding in the United States in 2005 was what?

14. The promises a couple makes to each other during the wedding ceremony are called what?

15. Often months before the wedding, the couple will create this at department stores to let people know which gifts, such as china and glassware, they would like to receive.

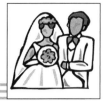

1. The future groom is the special guest at this party, usually held a day or two before the wedding.

    bachelor party

2. These judges, though not religious officials, often perform civil marriage ceremonies.

    justice of the peace

3. The white wedding gown is a tradition begun by this 19th-century Queen of England.

    Queen Victoria

4. This city in Nevada is the setting for thousands of civil wedding ceremonies each year.

    Las Vegas

5. Finish this common saying referring to what the bride-to-be should wear: "Something old, something new, . . ."

    something borrowed, something blue

6. This is another word for trousseau, the gifts that a bride's family typically gives to the family of the groom.

    dowry

7. This is what many grooms do as the married couple enters their home for the first time.

    carry the bride over the threshold

8. In many Asian countries, the wedding gown is this color, a "happy" color.

    red

9. The main member of the bride's wedding party is named this.

    maid of honor (matron of honor, if married)

10. If an unmarried woman catches this, it is said that she will be the next to be married.

    the bride's bouquet

11. If an unmarried man catches this, he, too, will be the next to be married!

    the bride's garter

12. A legal contract entered into by the couple prior to the wedding is called a what?

    prenuptial agreement

13. found that the average cost of a wedding in the United States in 2005 was what?

    $26,000

14. promises a couple makes to each other during the wedding ceremony are called what?

    wedding vows

15. Often months before the wedding, the couple will create this at department stores to let people know which gifts, such as china and glassware, they would like to receive.

    bridal registry

FACILITATOR: *This activity is sure to bring up a great deal of discussion. What do participants remember about their own wedding? Do they remember how much it cost? Who was in it? Do they still see these people today? What did they wear? What was served to eat and drink? If they had their wedding to do over again, would they do it differently? What do they think about the fact that weddings cost so much today? Is it worth it or would it be better to do things differently? Are there traditions, such as something borrowed, something blue, that have been passed down in their families?*

The Creative Spirit

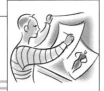

The works of great artists, whether chefs, painters, architects or other creative geniuses, inspire the imagination in all of us. The people listed below are creative icons—their creations have stood the test of time and continue to inspire new artistic styles today. Read the description of the person on the left and find the answer on the right.

____ 1. This creative woman has a dynasty all her own but is best known for her creativity in homemaking, cooking, and her television show " . . . Living."

____ 2. One of the most famous architects of all time, this man is noted for his "organic architecture" and introduction of open floor plans before his death in 1959.

____ 3. This renowned chef is known for his study of the relationship between food and culture and after his death left a legacy of food, including a foundation in his name and a culinary school at his home.

____ 4. This French woman revolutionized fashion in the early 1900s, but is perhaps best known for her signature "No. 5" perfume.

____ 5. Known as the "painter of light," this artist's paintings are often serene city or landscape scenes with glowing highlights.

____ 6. Known for his signature fashion line "Polo," this designer also has a large collection of vintage cars.

____ 7. This female architect is famous for designing Hearst Castle, the Los Angeles Examiner building, and her arts and crafts style architecture.

____ 8. Known for his Impressionist style, this famed artist is renowned for his series of over 250 paintings of water lilies.

____ 9. Widely recognized as a renaissance man and one of the greatest painters of all time, this man is most famous for his work of art, the Mona Lisa.

____ 10. Widely regarded as the world's greatest male ballet dancer, this Russian born performer has also starred in movies and television shows.

____ 11. This famous chef and television personality is known for introducing the art of French cooking to America.

____ 12. This composer is known for his theater hits such as "Memory" from the *Cats* production and "Music of the Night" from the *Phantom of the Opera*.

____ 13. Famous for his works of art such as the Campbell's Soup can, this controversial artist was also known for his underground films in the 1960s.

____ 14. One of the most famous opera singers in history, this Italian tenor was also known for his humanitarian works.

____ 15. As one of the pioneers of modern dance, this female dancer and choreographer is regarded as one of the greatest artists of the 20th century.

a. Andrew Lloyd Weber

b. Coco Chanel

c. Ralph Lauren

d. Mikhail Baryshnikov

e. Leonardo da Vinci

f. Martha Stewart

g. James Beard

h. Martha Graham

i. Claude Monet

j. Andy Warhol

k. Thomas Kinkade

l. Luciano Pavarotti

m. Julia Morgan

n. Frank Lloyd Wright

o. Julia Child

The Creative Spirit ANSWER SHEET

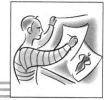

1. This creative woman has a dynasty all her own but is best known for her creativity in homemaking, cooking, and her television show " . . . Living."

    f.   **Martha Stewart**

2. One of the most famous architects of all time, this man is noted for his "organic architecture" and introduction of open floor plans before his death in 1959.

    n.   **Frank Lloyd Wright**

3. This renowned chef is known for his study of the relationship between food and culture and after his death left a legacy of food, including a foundation in his name and a culinary school at his home.

    g.   **James Beard**

4. This French woman revolutionized fashion in the early 1900s, but is perhaps best known for her signature "No. 5" perfume.

    b.   **Coco Chanel**

5. Known as the "painter of light," this artist's paintings are often serene city or landscape scenes with glowing highlights.

    k.   **Thomas Kinkade**

6. Known for his signature fashion line "Polo," this designer also has a large collection of vintage cars.

    c.   **Ralph Lauren**

7. This female architect is famous for designing Hearst Castle, the Los Angeles Examiner building, and her arts and crafts style architecture.

    m.   **Julia Morgan**

8. Known for his Impressionist style, this famed artist is renowned for his series of over 250 paintings of water lilies.

    i.   **Claude Monet**

9. Widely recognized as a renaissance man and one of the greatest painters of all time, this man is most famous for his work of art, the Mona Lisa.

    e.   **Leonardo da Vinci**

10. Widely regarded as the world's greatest male ballet dancer, this Russian born performer has also starred in movies and television shows.

    d.   **Mikhail Baryshnikov**

11. This famous chef and television personality is known for introducing the art of French cooking to America.

    o.   **Julia Child**

12. This composer is known for his theater hits such as "Memory" from the *Cats* production and "Music of the Night" from the *Phantom of the Opera.*

    a.   **Andrew Lloyd Weber**

13. Famous for his works of art such as the Campbell's Soup can, this controversial artist was also known for his underground films in the 1960s.

    j.   **Andy Warhol**

14. One of the most famous opera singers in history, this Italian tenor was also known for his humanitarian works.

    l.   **Luciano Pavarotti**

15. As one of the pioneers of modern dance, this female dancer and choreographer is regarded as one of the greatest artists of the 20th century.

    h.   **Martha Graham**

FACILITATOR: *The creative arts stimulate the senses. If possible, bring in samples of the artists' works to really see, hear, touch, taste, and feel them. Encourage conversation with the following questions: Are you a fan of any of these artists? Why or why not? Why do you think that many artists' lives are filled with controversy? Have you ever seen a performance or viewed any pieces from these artists? What other creative people could be listed here?*

Distinguished Women

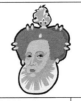

In the People section of this book, many famous women are mentioned. This activity focuses on some of the most distinguished women in history. Some of them have also been mentioned in other activities. All of them have made a difference! How many women can you name? If you need help with a name, see the list of women at the bottom of the next page.

1. This beloved first lady was one of the most active in American history. She helped draft the Universal Declaration of Human Rights and promoted the New Deal policies of her husband.

2. This social activist was best known for her role in the 19th-century women's rights movement. She fought for women's right to vote. Her face now adorns a dollar coin.

3. Nicknamed the "Maid of Orleans," this French woman rescued France from defeat during the 100 Years' War with England. She was burned at the stake.

4. This British Prime Minister served from 1979 until 1990 and was the first woman to lead a major party in the United Kingdom. She was nicknamed the "Iron Lady" due to her image of having a steadfast, iron-like character.

5. This woman, beloved by all, was considered by many to be the greatest all-around female athlete of all time. She excelled in golf, basketball, and track and field.

6. This supreme leader of Egypt had a liaison with Julius Caesar and, after his death, with Mark Antony. She was the last pharaoh of ancient Egypt. It is said that she took her own life by allowing an asp to bite her. Many famous works have been written of her life.

7. This woman was crowned Queen of England in 1838 and she reigned for 63 years, the longest in British history. Under her rule, the United Kingdom became the world leader in the 1800s. The era of her reign was famously named after her.

8. This Roman Catholic nun, nicknamed The "Saint of the Gutters," founded a religious order called the Missionaries of Charity. She received the 1979 Nobel Peace Prize.

9. This aviator was the first to fly solo over the Atlantic Ocean, eventually disappearing over the Pacific Ocean. She was the first woman to receive the Distinguished Flying Cross.

10. This famous American novelist was a bitter enemy of the South. She is best known for her anti-slavery novel, *Uncle Tom's Cabin*. Upon meeting her, Abraham Lincoln said, "So you're the little woman who wrote the book that started this great war!"

11. This distinguished American nurse was a great humanitarian and was best known for organizing the Red Cross in 1881.

12. This woman is one of America's most gifted poets. She wrote more than 1,700 poems, but did not wish to publish any of them. One of her best known is "Success Is Counted Sweetest."

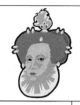

13. This young Holocaust victim lived in hiding with her family and four friends in Amsterdam during the German occupation. The diary entries she wrote while in hiding were published as the very famous *The Diary of a Young Girl*.

14. This amazing woman, left blind and deaf by an illness at 19 months old, went on to become an advocate for people with disabilities. She spent much of her life raising funds to help people with vision loss. Anne Sullivan was her teacher and friend for 49 years.

15. This woman, nicknamed "Lady with the Lamp," pioneered the profession of nursing. She brought sanitation to war-time nursing.

16. This California politician became the first female Speaker of the House in 2006.

17. This "Queen of Comedy" was thought by many to be the best female comedienne in movie and television history. She was married for a long while to a Cuban bandleader.

18. This American novelist wrote *Little Women*, which has been read by, among others, many, many young girls. The book was partially based on her young life growing up with three sisters.

19. This Shoshone woman accompanied Lewis and Clark on their expedition from North Dakota to the Pacific Ocean in the early 1800s and was very instrumental in their successful journey, serving as both a guide and an interpreter.

20. This astronaut was the first American female in space on the shuttle Challenger.

21. Named by the U.S. Congress as the "Mother of the Modern-Day Civil Rights Movement," this woman became famous for refusing to give up her seat to a white man on a Montgomery, Alabama, bus in 1955. Thus began the Montgomery bus boycott against racial segregation.

22. This judge became the first female member of the Supreme Court.

23. This woman was born a slave in the early 1800s, but went on to become an abolitionist, leading the Underground Railroad and over 300 slaves to freedom.

Choices: Lucille Ball – Helen Keller – Sandra Day O'Connor – Queen Victoria – Eleanor Roosevelt – Clara Barton – Amelia Earhart – Susan B. Anthony – Emily Dickinson – Harriet Tubman – Anne Frank – Margaret Thatcher – Harriet Beecher Stowe – Mother Teresa – Louisa May Alcott – Rosa Parks – Cleopatra – Joan of Arc – Sally Ride – Sakajawea – "Babe" Didrikson Zaharias – Florence Nightingale – Nancy Pelosi

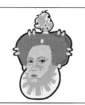

Distinguished Women ANSWER SHEET

1. This beloved first lady was one of the most active in American history. She helped draft the Universal Declaration of Human Rights and promoted the New Deal policies of her husband.
   Eleanor Roosevelt

2. This social activist was best known for her role in the 19th-century women's rights movement. She fought for women's right to vote. Her face now adorns a dollar coin.
   Susan B. Anthony

3. Nicknamed the "Maid of Orleans," this French woman rescued France from defeat during the 100 Years' War with England. She was burned at the stake.
   Joan of Arc

4. This British Prime Minister served from 1979 until 1990 and was the first woman to lead a major party in the United Kingdom. She was nicknamed the "Iron Lady" due to her image of having a steadfast, iron-like character.
   Margaret Thatcher

5. This woman, beloved by all, was considered by many to be the greatest all-around female athlete of all time. She excelled in golf, basketball, and track and field.
   "Babe" Didrikson Zaharias

6. This supreme leader of Egypt had a liaison with Julius Caesar and, after his death, with Mark Antony. She was the last pharaoh of ancient Egypt. It is said that she took her own life by allowing an asp to bite her. Many famous works have been written of her life.
   Cleopatra

7. This woman was crowned Queen of England in 1838 and she reigned for 63 years, the longest in British history. Under her rule, the United Kingdom became the world leader in the 1800s. The era of her reign was famously named after her.
   Queen Victoria

8. This Roman Catholic nun, nicknamed The "Saint of the Gutters," founded a religious order called the Missionaries of Charity. She received the 1979 Nobel Peace Prize.
   Mother Teresa

9. This aviator was the first to fly solo over the Atlantic Ocean, eventually disappearing over the Pacific Ocean. She was the first woman to receive the Distinguished Flying Cross.
   Amelia Earhart

10. This famous American novelist was a bitter enemy of the South. She is best known for her anti-slavery novel, *Uncle Tom's Cabin*. Upon meeting her, Abraham Lincoln said, "So you're the little woman who wrote the book that started this great war!"
    Harriet Beecher Stowe

11. This distinguished American nurse was a great humanitarian and was best known for organizing the Red Cross in 1881.
    Clara Barton

12. This woman is one of America's most gifted poets. She wrote more than 1,700 poems, but did not wish to publish any of them. One of her best known is "Success Is Counted Sweetest."
    Emily Dickinson

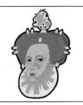

13. This young Holocaust victim lived in hiding with her family and four friends in Amsterdam during the German occupation. The diary entries she wrote while in hiding were published as the very famous *The Diary of a Young Girl*.
    Anne Frank

14. This amazing woman, left blind and deaf by an illness at 19 months old, went on to become an advocate for people with disabilities. She spent much of her life raising funds to help people with vision loss. Anne Sullivan was her teacher and friend for 49 years.
    Helen Keller

15. This woman, nicknamed "Lady with the Lamp," pioneered the profession of nursing. She brought sanitation to war-time nursing.
    Florence Nightingale

16. This California politician became the first female Speaker of the House in 2006.
    Nancy Pelosi

17. This "Queen of Comedy" was thought by many to be the best female comedienne in movie and television history. She was married for a long while to a Cuban bandleader.
    Lucille Ball

18. This American novelist wrote *Little Women*, which has been read by, among others, many, many young girls. The book was partially based on her young life growing up with three sisters.
    Louisa May Alcott

19. This Shoshone woman accompanied Lewis and Clark on their expedition from North Dakota to the Pacific Ocean in the early 1800s and was very instrumental in their successful journey, serving as both a guide and an interpreter.
    Sakajawea

20. This astronaut was the first American female in space on the shuttle Challenger.
    Sally Ride

21. Named by the U.S. Congress as the "Mother of the Modern-Day Civil Rights Movement," this woman became famous for refusing to give up her seat to a white man on a Montgomery, Alabama, bus in 1955. Thus began the Montgomery bus boycott against racial segregation.
    Rosa Parks

22. This judge became the first female member of the Supreme Court.
    Sandra Day O'Connor

23. This woman was born a slave in the early 1800s, but went on to become an abolitionist, leading the Underground Railroad and over 300 slaves to freedom.
    Harriet Tubman

FACILITATOR: This activity lends itself to a variety of discussions. First of all, it's important to discuss each woman and her contributions. What difference did each woman make in the lives of women today and in the past? Do participants agree that these are all women who deserve the term "distinguished"? Ask why it is that so few women are included in history books. Is this changing? Which famous women are making a difference in the world today? Will they be included in the history books of tomorrow? Will there ever be equal numbers of women as there are men in history books? The discussion, if desired, could then go into whether or not men and women are truly equal. Why or why not? If participants were to be invited to spend the day with one woman in history, who would they choose and why?

Expressions Related to People

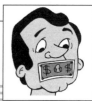

The English language is full of sayings that do not make literal sense. Phrases such as "grab the bull by the horns" mean something completely different than their true translation. The sayings in this worksheet are no exception. All of the sayings (and answers) are related to people. Read the description on the left and match it with its meaning on the right.

___ 1. A person who acts all knowing or who shows off his or her knowledge.

___ 2. To speak angrily to someone.

___ 3. A type of belief or proverb passed from generation to generation that is not necessarily true.

___ 4. A child who is similar to a parent.

___ 5. A person who is genuine is said to be

___ 6. A person who tries to be seen as having the same material wealth as his or her neighbors.

___ 7. A renaissance man or a person who is skilled in many areas.

___ 8. A person who spends his or her money unwisely will lose it quickly, is the meaning of this saying.

___ 9. A task that is exceptionally easy.

___ 10. A person who is very wealthy.

___ 11. A woman who has been in many weddings but who has never.

___ 12. A person who sleeps very soundly.

___ 13. Someone who tells mistruths often and without remorse.

___ 14. A person in the passenger seat who gives the driver advice on how to maneuver the vehicle.

___ 15. A person who uses extremely foul language.

___ 16. To give up or surrender.

___ 17. Something that is needed or wanted.

___ 18. An ordinary, typical person.

a. a man of means

b. the real McCoy

c. average Joe

d. backseat driver

e. smart Aleck

f. just what the Dr. ordered

g. barefaced liar

h. swear like a sailor

i. sleep like a baby

j. keep up with the Jones's

k. read them the riot act

l. chip off the old block

m. Jack of all trades

n. a fool and his money are soon parted

o. always a bridesmaid, never a bride

p. old wives' tale

q. cry uncle

r. child's play

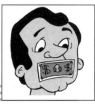

1. A person who acts all knowing or who shows off his or her knowledge.

   e. smart Aleck

2. To speak angrily to someone.

   k. read them the riot act

3. A type of belief or proverb passed from generation to generation that is not necessarily true.

   p. old wives' tale

4. A child who is similar to a parent.

   l. chip off the old block

5. A person who is genuine.

   b. the real McCoy

6. A person who tries to be seen as having the same material wealth as his or her neighbors.

   j. keep up with the Jones's

7. A renaissance man or a person who is skilled in many areas.

   m. Jack of all trades

8. A person who spends his or her money unwisely will lose it quickly, is the meaning of this saying.

   n. a fool and his money are soon parted

9. A task that is exceptionally easy.

   r. child's play

10. A person who is very wealthy.

    a. a man of means

11. A woman who has been in many weddings but who has never married.

    o. always a bridesmaid, never a bride

12. A person who sleeps very soundly.

    i. sleep like a baby

13. Someone who tells mistruths often and without remorse.

    g. barefaced liar

14. A person in the passenger seat who gives the driver advice on how to maneuver the vehicle.

    d. backseat driver

15. A person who uses extremely foul language.

    h. swear like a sailor

16. To give up or surrender.

    q. cry uncle

17. Something that is needed or wanted.

    f. just what the Dr. ordered

18. An ordinary, typical person.

    c. average Joe

FACILITATOR: *There are many expressions related to people that are not listed. Can the group think of more? How about expressions with places? How do participants think these expressions came about? What expressions do people in the group use regularly? Which expressions could be considered "overused"?*

Famous Scandals

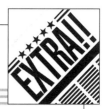

Scandals seem to be a staple of the political and entertainment world. Listed below are the descriptions of many well-known incidents where people had the "wool pulled over their eyes." Match the description on the left with the name on the right.

____ 1. In the 1950s, it was revealed that several popular television quiz shows were secretly rigged by producers.

____ 2. Orson Wells directed an adaptation of this novel that aired on October 30, 1968, causing many to believe that an actual alien invasion was taking place in the United States.

____ 3. This well-known political scandal took place in 1972 in Washington, DC, and led to the resignation of President Nixon.

____ 4. In this famous archeological hoax, pieces of bone believed to be that of an early human were, over 40 years later, discovered to be that of a modern man and an orangutan.

____ 5. This Texas-based energy company was once considered one of the most innovative, successful companies to work for, until it was forced into bankruptcy by a major accounting fraud.

____ 6. This famous televangelist and minister was convicted of accounting fraud for misusing hundreds of thousands of dollars in donations given to his popular ministry in the 1980s.

____ 7. During the Reagan Administration, this political scandal involved selling weapons to Iran and using the profits to fund anti-communist rebels.

____ 8. In the 1990s, this famous filmmaker came under scrutiny for having a relationship with his long-time girl-friend's adopted daughter, whom he later married.

____ 9. This famous scandal took place under President Harding in 1921 and involved a navy oil reserve being secretly leased to a private company.

____ 10. The 1919 World Series resulted in this famous baseball scandal involving eight players who attempted to "fix" the game.

____ 11. In this Hollywood scandal, actors Debbie Reynolds and Eddie Fisher ended their marriage when it was revealed that Fisher fell in love with whom?

____ 12. In 1875, it was revealed that a group of distillers and public officials were stealing the proceeds of over-inflated taxes on liquor.

____ 13. Some say that there are still sightings of this famous rock star who died in 1977, leading many to say that he faked his own death.

a. Enron

b. Elvis Presley

c. Black Sox Scandal

d. Quiz Show Scandals

e. Iran Contra Affair

f. Watergate

g. The Whiskey Ring

h. Elizabeth Taylor

i. *War of the Worlds*

j. Piltdown Man

k. Jim Bakker

l. Woody Allen

m. Teapot Dome

1. In the 1950s, it was revealed that several popular television quiz shows were secretly rigged by producers.

    d. Quiz Show Scandals

2. Orson Wells directed an adaptation of this novel that aired on October 30, 1968, causing many to believe that an actual alien invasion was taking place in the United States.

    i. *War of the Worlds*

3. This well-known political scandal took place in 1972 in Washington, DC, and led to the resignation of President Nixon.

    f. Watergate

4. In this famous archeological hoax, pieces of bone believed to be that of an early human were, over 40 years later, discovered to be that of a modern man and an orangutan.

    j. Piltdown man

5. This Texas-based energy company was once considered one of the most innovative, successful companies to work for, until it was forced into bankruptcy by a major accounting fraud.

    a. Enron

6. This famous televangelist and minister was convicted of accounting fraud for misusing hundreds of thousands of dollars in donations given to his popular ministry in the 1980s.

    k. Jim Bakker

7. During the Reagan Administration, this political scandal involved selling weapons to Iran and using the profits to fund anti-communist rebels.

    e. Iran Contra Affair

8. In the 1990s, this famous filmmaker came under scrutiny for having a relationship with his long-time girlfriend's adopted daughter, whom he later married.

    l. Woody Allen

9. This famous scandal took place under President Harding in 1921 and involved a navy oil reserve being secretly leased to a private company.

    m. Teapot Dome

10. The 1919 World Series resulted in this famous baseball scandal involving eight players who attempted to "fix" the game.

    c. Black Sox Scandal

11. In this Hollywood scandal, actors Debbie Reynolds and Eddie Fisher ended their marriage when it was revealed that Fisher fell in love with whom?

    h. Elizabeth Taylor

12. In 1875, it was revealed that a group of distillers and public officials were stealing the proceeds of over-inflated taxes on liquor.

    g. The Whiskey Ring

13. Some say that there are still sightings of this famous rock star who died in 1977, leading many to say that he faked his own death.

    b. Elvis Presley

FACILITATOR: *This sheet is sure to bring up discussion on right versus wrong. What does the group think about each of these scandals? Were any of these incidents justified? Which is more detrimental, a Hollywood scandal or a po-litical scandal? What role does/did the media play in these scandals or current scandals? Can the group think of any additional scandals not mentioned here?*

Famous Child Actors

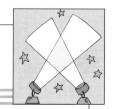

Many actors and actresses began their career as young children. Some were famous for only a short time while others enjoyed popularity that lasted well into their adult years. Below is a list of children famous for their roles in television or film. Match the description of the child on the left with the name on the right.

___ 1. Known for her standout role in the 1944 movie *National Velvet*, this child star is also famous for her many husbands as an adult.

    a. Our Gang

___ 2. This child star is known for both her role in the 1962 film *The Miracle Worker*, for which she received an Academy Award, and for the television series named after her.

    b. Mary Pickford

___ 3. Known for playing Opie Taylor on *The Andy Griffith Show*, this child actor grew up to be an award-winning film director.

    c. Jackie Coogan

___ 4. At the age of 10, this child actress became the youngest person to win an Academy Award for her role in the 1973 film *Paper Moon*.

    d. Elizabeth Taylor

___ 5. Known as "the girl with the curls," this child actress was one of the most prominent figures in the silent film industry.

    e. Judy Garland

___ 6. This actress has performed in dozens of movies, but is best known for her performances in *Pollyanna* (1960) and *The Parent Trap* (1961).

    f. Angela/Veronica Cartwright

___ 7. The career of this child actor has spanned over 80 years, but he may best be known for his string of successful Andy Hardy films with Judy Garland.

    g. Hayley Mills

___ 8. This child actress is famous for her role as Dorothy in *The Wizard of Oz* and is considered one of the greatest female stars of all time.

    h. Ron Howard

___ 9. This series of short films in the 1930s featured the antics of a variety of child actors, but is best known for the comedy of Spanky, Alfalfa, and Buckwheat.

___ 10. Known for his role alongside Charlie Chaplin in the 1921 film *The Kid* this actor was also famous for his page boy–style haircut.

    i. Mickey Rooney

___ 11. This actress made many films both as a child and an adult and is known for her role in the 1947 movie *Miracle on 34th Street*.

    j. Patty Duke

___ 12. This award-winning actress first appeared on stage at the age of 2 and is most well known for her roles in films such as *Mary Poppins* and *The Sound of Music*.

    k. Tatum O'Neal

___ 13. This well-known actor is most famous for his role as Beaver in the well loved 1950s and 1960s series *Leave It To Beaver*.

    l. Jerry Mathers

___ 14. These two sisters are famous for their film and television appearances in the 1950s. One starred in the television series *Lost In Space* and the other had a regular role in *Leave It To Beaver*.

    m. Julie Andrews

___ 15. There are several children (real or character) known for advertising a product. Can you name at least three?

    n. Natalie Wood

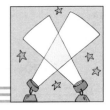

1. Known for her standout role in the 1944 movie *National Velvet*, this child star is also famous for her many husbands as an adult.

2. This child star is known for both her role in the 1962 film *The Miracle Worker*, for which she received an Academy Award, and for the television series named after her.

3. Known for playing Opie Taylor on *The Andy Griffith Show*, this child actor grew up to be an award-winning film director.

4. At the age of 10, this child actress became the youngest person to win an Academy Award for her role in the 1973 film *Paper Moon*.

5. Known as "the girl with the curls," this child actress was one of the most prominent figures in the silent film industry.

6. This actress has performed in dozens of movies, but is best known for her performances in *Pollyanna* (1960) and *The Parent Trap* (1961).

7. The career of this child actor has spanned over 80 years, but he may best be known for his string of successful Andy Hardy films with Judy Garland.

8. This child actress is famous for her role as Dorothy in *The Wizard of Oz* and is considered one of the greatest female stars of all time.

9. This series of short films in the 1930s featured the antics of a variety of child actors, but is best known for the comedy of Spanky, Alfalfa, and Buckwheat.

10. Known for his role alongside Charlie Chaplin in the 1921 film *The Kid* this actor was also famous for his page boy–style haircut.

11. This actress made many films both as a child and an adult and is known for her role in the 1947 movie *Miracle on 34th Street*.

12. This award-winning actress first appeared on stage at the age of 2 and is most well known for her roles in films such as *Mary Poppins* and *The Sound of Music*.

13. This well-known actor is most famous for his role as Beaver in the well loved 1950s and 1960s series *Leave It To Beaver*.

14. These two sisters are famous for their film and television appearances in the 1950s. One starred in the television series *Lost In Space* and the other had a regular role in *Leave It To Beaver*.

15. There are several children (real or character) known for advertising a product. Can you name at least three?

d. **Elizabeth Taylor**

j. **Patty Duke**

h. **Ron Howard**

k. **Tatum O'Neal**

b. **Mary Pickford**

g. **Hayley Mills**

i. **Mickey Rooney**

e. **Judy Garland**

a. **Our Gang**

c. **Jackie Coogan**

n. **Natalie Wood**

m. **Julie Andrews**

l. **Jerry Mathers**

f. **Angela/Veronica Cartwright**

Gerber Baby, Morton Salt Girl, Coppertone Girl, Wendy's Girl, Willy Wonka, Mikey (Life Cereal), Doublemint Twins, Alfred E. Newman (*MAD Magazine*)

FACILITATOR: *This worksheet is sure to bring up discussion on favorite childhood actors and actresses. How many of these movies have you seen? Did you have any favorite child actors? How does Hollywood treat young stars? Were young stars given too much freedom in Hollywood's golden age? How about today? What does it take to have a successful acting career as a child and an adult? What level of involvement should parents have in a child actor's professional life?*

Famous Couples

There have been many famous couples throughout history, famous for both their relationships and their careers. Some have been married. Some simply had love affairs. Some are fictional. Others are real. Based on the clues given, how many of the following couples can you name?

1. This romantic couple were the Italian stars of one of Shakespeare's most famous plays set in Verona, Italy.

2. Their story, told in the Bible in the book of Genesis, takes place in the Garden of Eden.

3. This man and woman married after their love affair caused him to relinquish the throne in England.

4. Her ugly stepsisters could not keep this fictional couple from finding each other, thanks to her fairy godmother and the fit of a glass slipper.

5. This couple played themselves on their comedy show, which premiered in the 1950s. They were one of the most famous comedy teams ever.

6   This fictional couple consisted of a giant gorilla and his improbable love interest.

7. This very famous couple began their relationship when both were filming *Cleopatra*. They later married, divorced, and then married again.

8. This man, who is "faster than a speeding bullet," and his girlfriend are both reporters for the *Daily Planet*.

9. This couple were the ever-popular stars of *Gone with the Wind*.

10. Johnny Weissmuller played the male role in this fictional African jungle couple who had a pet chimp named Cheeta.

11. This fictional couple were part of the Merry Men and spent a great deal of time guarding Sherwood Forest.

12. *Walk the Line* was a movie made about this entertainment industry couple. The man was known as the "man in black."

13. This blonde sex symbol and baseball player were married just short of a year, but had a lasting friendship. He left red roses at her grave regularly for 20 years after her death.

14. Even though this Hollywood couple never married, they had a 27-year love affair, both on screen and off. Both were Academy Award winners.

15. This Academy Award–winning American actress and the Prince of Monaco were married in what many called "the wedding of the century."

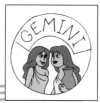

Famous Couples ANSWER SHEET

1. This romantic couple were the Italian stars of one of Shakespeare's most famous plays set in Verona, Italy.
    Romeo and Juliet

2. Their story, told in the Bible in the book of Genesis, takes place in the Garden of Eden.
    Adam and Eve

3. This man and woman married after their love affair caused him to relinquish the throne in England.
    Edward VIII and Wallis Simpson

4. Her ugly stepsisters could not keep this fictional couple from finding each other, thanks to her fairy godmother and the fit of a glass slipper.
    Cinderella and Prince Charming

5. This couple played themselves on their comedy show, which premiered in the 1950s. They were one of the most famous comedy teams ever.
    George Burns and Gracie Allen

6   This fictional couple consisted of a giant gorilla and his improbable love interest.
    King Kong and Faye Ray

7. This very famous couple began their relationship when both were filming *Cleopatra*. They later married, divorced, and then married again.
    Richard Burton and Elizabeth Taylor

8. This man, who is "faster than a speeding bullet," and his girlfriend are both reporters for the *Daily Planet*.
    Superman and Lois Lane

9. This couple were the ever-popular stars of *Gone with the Wind*.
    Rhett Butler and Scarlett O'Hara

10. Johnny Weissmuller played the male role in this fictional African jungle couple who had a pet chimp named Cheeta.
    Tarzan and Jane

11. This fictional couple were part of the Merry Men and spent a great deal of time guarding Sherwood Forest.
    Robin Hood and Maid Marian

12. *Walk the Line* was a movie made about this entertainment industry couple. The man was known as the "man in black."
    Johnny Cash and June Carter Cash

13. This blonde sex symbol and baseball player were married just short of a year, but had a lasting friendship. He left red roses at her grave regularly for 20 years after her death.
    Joe DiMaggio and Marilyn Monroe

14. Even though this Hollywood couple never married, they had a 27-year love affair, both on screen and off. Both were Academy Award winners.
    Katherine Hepburn and Spencer Tracy

15. This Academy Award–winning American actress and the Prince of Monaco were married in what many called "the wedding of the century."
    Grace Kelly and Prince Rainier

FACILITATOR: *Ask participants what they know about these couples. What made them famous as couples? Were they well respected? Which other famous couples can participants identify? Cleopatra and both Mark Antony and Caeser, Guinevere and Lancelot, Porgy and Bess, Samson and Delilah, Bonnie and Clyde? What do they believe it takes to have a truly lasting relationship? What characteristics are necessary?*

Famous "Doubles"

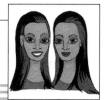

Many people have first and last names beginning with the same letter of the alphabet. Some were born with these names. Others changed either one or both to create more memorable or marketable names. The following people all have first and last names beginning with the letters indicated. How many can you name?

1. Her low, husky voice was a trademark of this Swedish film star who began in silent films but later also made it big in talking pictures.
    G_____G_____

2. "Won't You Come Home?" is asked of this man in the very popular song with a title the same as his name.
    B_____B_____

3. This Italian reportedly "discovered" the United States.
    C_____C_____

4. This Hungarian magician was perhaps most famous for his acts of "escapism."
    H_____H_____

5. This famous American photographer was best known for his black and white photos. He took some especially famous pictures of national parks, including Yosemite.
    A_____A_____

6. This 19th-century American poet is best known for his collection of poems entitled *Leaves of Grass*.
    W_____W_____

7. This musical film and stage star had many leading roles, including *South Pacific*, *Peter Pan*, and *The Sound of Music*.
    M_____M_____

8. The "Tennessee Waltz" was one of the most famous songs recorded by this well-known pop singer of the 1950s and beyond.
    P_____P_____

9. "Que sera, sera" was a song made famous by this 1950s perky blonde actress and singer. She starred in many romantic comedies. One of the best known is *Pillow Talk* with Rock Hudson.
    D_____D_____

10. This 30th president of the United States was known as "Silent Cal."
    C_____C_____

11. This 20th-century Spanish painter and sculptor was most famous for first using Cubism, a form of art using geometric shapes.
    P_____P_____

12. This powerful centerfielder played for the New York Yankees his entire career in the 1950s and '60s. Many of his records remain valid today.
    M_____M_____

13. This 28th president of the United States kept the country out of World War I until it seemed no longer possible in 1917. He introduced the League of Nations as a means of ending the war.
    W_____W_____

14. This lady was an actress and gossip columnist in the first half of the 20th century. She had a famous long-standing feud with Louella Parsons.
    H_____H_____

15. This 20th-century American newscaster and broadcaster invented the gossip column. He was both popular and very controversial in the world of radio.
    W_____W_____

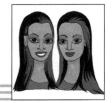

1. Her low, husky voice was a trademark of this Swedish film star who began in silent films but later also made it big in talking pictures.
   Greta Garbo

2. "Won't You Come Home?" is asked of this man in the very popular song with a title the same as his name.
   Bill Bailey

3. This Italian reportedly "discovered" the United States.
   Christopher Columbus

4. This Hungarian magician was perhaps most famous for his acts of "escapism."
   Harry Houdini

5. This famous American photographer was best known for his black and white photos. He took some especially famous pictures of national parks, including Yosemite.
   Ansel Adams

6. This 19th-century American poet is best known for his collection of poems entitled *Leaves of Grass*.
   Walt Whitman

7. This musical film and stage star had many leading roles, including *South Pacific*, *Peter Pan*, and *The Sound of Music*.
   Mary Martin

8. The "Tennessee Waltz" was one of the most famous songs recorded by this well-known pop singer of the 1950s and beyond.
   Patty Page

9. "Que sera, sera" was a song made famous by this 1950s perky blonde actress and singer. She starred in many romantic comedies. One of the best known is *Pillow Talk* with Rock Hudson.
   Doris Day

10. This 30th president of the United States was known as "Silent Cal."
    Calvin Coolidge

11. This 20th-century Spanish painter and sculptor was most famous for first using Cubism, a form of art using geometric shapes.
    Pablo Picasso

12. This powerful centerfielder played for the New York Yankees his entire career in the 1950s and '60s. Many of his records remain valid today.
    Mickey Mantle

13. This 28th president of the United States kept the country out of World War I until it seemed no longer possible in 1917. He introduced the League of Nations as a means of ending the war.
    Woodrow Wilson

14. This lady was an actress and gossip columnist in the first half of the 20th century. She had a famous long-standing feud with Louella Parsons.
    Hedda Hopper

15. This 20th-century American newscaster and broadcaster invented the gossip column. He was both popular and very controversial in the world of radio.
    Walter Winchell

FACILITATOR: *Ask participants which of these people they consider most famous. Who are others with both first and last names that begin with the same letter? You might want to go through the alphabet to come up with ideas. Possibilities include Barry Bonds, Robert Redford, Danny DeVito, Claudette Colbert, Sam Spade, George Gobel, Bugs Bunny, and Sylvester Stallone. Another topic of conversation might be why people change their names. Do they not like their names? Do they think another name will make them more popular? Do they change their name in an attempt to leave the past behind?*

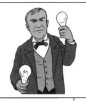

Famous People and the Occupations that Made Them So

The following people were all famous—and sometimes rich—on account of their occupations. Match the occupation on the left with the famous person who worked in that occupation on the right.

___ 1. Orchestra conductor

___ 2. Suffragette

___ 3. Marine biologist

___ 4. Photographer

___ 5. Silversmith

___ 6. Gossip columnist

___ 7. Outlaw

___ 8. Nurse

___ 9. Poet

___ 10. Astronomer

___ 11. Cellist

___ 12. Detective

___ 13. Spy

___ 14. Journalist and writer

___ 15. World War II General

___ 16. Inventor

___ 17. Scientist

___ 18. Sculptor

___ 19. Newscaster

___ 20. Director

a. Galileo Galilei

b. Marie Curie

c. Ansel Adams

d. Mata Hari

e. Sherlock Holmes

f. Thomas Edison

g. Leonard Bernstein

h. Clara Barton

i. Walter Brinkley

j. Michelangelo

k. Jacques Cousteau

l. Elizabeth Cady Stanton

m. Walt Whitman

n. Samuel Clemens

o. Hedda Hopper

p. Pablo Casals

q. George Patton Jr.

r. Paul Revere

s. George Lucas

t. Jesse James

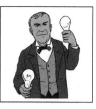

Famous People and the Occupations that Made Them So
ANSWER SHEET

1.	Orchestra conductor	g.	**Leonard Bernstein**
2.	Suffragette	l.	**Elizabeth Cady Stanton**
3.	Marine biologist	k.	**Jacques Cousteau**
4.	Photographer	c.	**Ansel Adams**
5.	Silversmith	r.	**Paul Revere**
6.	Gossip columnist	o.	**Hedda Hopper**
7.	Outlaw	t.	**Jesse James**
8.	Nurse	h.	**Clara Barton**
9.	Poet	m.	**Walt Whitman**
10.	Astronomer	a.	**Galileo Galilei**
11.	Cellist	p.	**Pablo Casals**
12.	Detective	e.	**Sherlock Holmes**
13.	Spy	d.	**Mata Hari**
14.	Journalist and writer	n.	**Samuel Clemens**
15.	World War II General	q.	**George Patton Jr.**
16.	Inventor	f.	**Thomas Edison**
17.	Scientist	b.	**Marie Curie**
18.	Sculptor	j.	**Michelangelo**
19.	Newscaster	i.	**Walter Brinkley**
20.	Director	s.	**George Lucas**

FACILITATOR: *After completing this activity would be a good time to talk about the particpants' occupations. What was their first job? Their last? Their favorite? Which of the occupations of these famous people would they like to have had? Which of these people do they especially admire? Are there particular things that made these people famous?*

Famous People Defined by Their Hairstyles and Hats

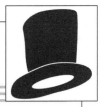

Attention to hairstyles began thousands of years ago, as exemplified by Cleopatra. Over the years, many famous people have been defined, at least in part, by their hairstyles. The same can be said for hats, which have also been around for thousands of years. They were most likely first used as head coverings to protect against the elements. Can you name the person often identified with the following hair, hairstyle, or hat? Match the person from the right column to the clue on the left.

___ 1.	Ringlet curls	a. Mary Tyler Moore
___ 2.	Towering hats made of fruit	b. Laurel and Hardy
___ 3.	Bald	c. Shirley Temple
___ 4.	Top hat	d. Spanky of Our Gang
___ 5.	Platinum blonde	e. Davy Crockett
___ 6.	Pillbox hat	f. Abraham Lincoln
___ 7.	A "girl next door" flip	g. W. C. Fields
___ 8.	Panama hat	h. Sherlock Holmes
___ 9.	Peak-a-boo or the flapper look	i. Carmen Miranda
___ 10.	Coonskin cap	j. Minnie Pearl
___ 11.	Side-parted finger waves	k. Winston Churchill
___ 12.	Deerstalker or tweed hat	l. Lucille Ball
___ 13.	Long hair for men, made famous by this "quartet"	m. Marilyn Monroe
___ 14.	Bowler hat	n. Jean Harlow
___ 15.	The wedge, made famous by this ice-skater	o. Jackie Kennedy
___ 16.	A hat with a $1.98 price tag	p. Dorothy Hamill
___ 17.	Stove-pipe hat	q. Clara Bow
___ 18.	Flaming red hair	r. Beatles
___ 19.	Beanie	s. Yul Brenner

Famous People Defined by Their Hairstyles and Hats

ANSWER SHEET

1.	Ringlet curls	c.	**Shirley Temple**
2.	Towering hats made of fruit	i.	**Carmen Miranda**
3.	Bald	s.	**Yul Brenner**
4.	Top hat	f.	**Abraham Lincoln**
5.	Platinum blonde	m.	**Marilyn Monroe**
6.	Pillbox hat	o.	**Jackie Kennedy**
7.	A "girl next door" flip	a.	**Mary Tyler Moore**
8.	Panama hat	k.	**Winston Churchill**
9.	Peak-a-boo or the flapper look	q.	**Clara Bow**
10.	Coonskin cap	e.	**Davy Crockett**
11.	Side-parted finger waves	n.	**Jean Harlow**
12.	Deerstalker or tweed hat	h.	**Sherlock Holmes**
13.	Long hair for men, made famous by this "quartet"	r.	**Beatles**
14.	Bowler hat	b.	**Laurel and Hardy**
15.	The wedge, made famous by this ice-skater	p.	**Dorothy Hamill**
16.	A hat with a $1.98 price tag	j.	**Minnie Pearl**
17.	Stove-pipe hat	g.	**W. C. Fields**
18.	Flaming red hair	l.	**Lucille Ball**
19.	Beanie	d.	**Spanky of Our Gang**

FACILITATOR: *This activity lends itself to bringing in different types of hats or maybe having everyone bring in their favorites. Discuss why these hats/hairstyles became famous. Do participants find them memorable? Which are their favorites? What is their favorite kind of hat? Favorite hairstyle? Favorite color of hair? If possible, bring in some pictures of the above people to get the conversation started. Regarding hats, why do participants think people wear hats? Has this changed over the years? Why don't as many people wear hats today?*

Famous Siblings

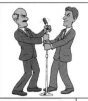

Throughout history, many siblings have all become famous in their own rights—some for doing things together, some for doing things on their own. The following brothers and sisters are all famous for a variety of reasons. Can you name these famous siblings?

1. These 3 Hungarian sisters were all actresses, but were probably best known for their multiple marriages—19 between the 3 of them!

2. This brother and sister were children of the 35th U.S. president. One of their most famous photographs was of them standing watching their father's funeral procession, the young boy saluting.

3. These boys were the sons, both on television and in real life, of Ozzie and Harriet.

4. These three English sisters of the 1800s were famous in literature. Their works, which include *Jane Eyre*, *Wuthering Heights*, and *Agnes Grey*, are still read by many today.

5. These brothers are credited with building the first successful airplane.

6. These four singing sisters were perhaps best known for their years on the *Lawrence Welk Show*.

7. These brothers from Biblical times are often thought to be the first two sons of Adam and Eve.

8. These five comedian brothers often acted in vaudeville, movies, and, later, television.

9. These three sisters sang pop songs in the 1950s and '60s. They first appeared on *Arthur Godfry's Talent Scouts* in 1952. They went on to sign a very lucrative deal with Coca Cola and advertised with them for many years.

10. These two brothers are often thought of as the founders of Rome.

11. These two brothers formed a music and comedy team, giving live performances and starring in their own television shows in the latter part of the 20th century. They were famous for folk songs and for "arguing" with each other during performances.

12. These identical twin girls both changed their names and wrote advice columns in various newspapers for many, many years.

13. In the 1930s, these three sisters became the first female vocal group to earn a Gold Record. They recorded such popular hits as "Don't Sit Under the Apple Tree," "I'll Be With You in Apple Blossom Time," and the "Beer Barrel Polka." They sang many of their songs with Bing Crosby.

14. These two British acting sisters have both won Academy Awards. One sister won her first award for her role as Melanie in *Gone with the Wind* and the other for her role in Alfred Hitchcock's *Suspicion*.

15. These two brothers and two sisters are the children of Queen Elizabeth II and Prince Phillip.

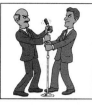

1. These 3 Hungarian sisters were all actresses, but were probably best known for their multiple marriages—19 between the 3 of them!
   Eva, Magda, and Zsa Zsa Gabor

2. This brother and sister were children of the 35th U.S. president. One of their most famous photographs was of them standing watching their father's funeral procession, the young boy saluting.
   Caroline and John Kennedy

3. These boys were the sons, both on television and in real life, of Ozzie and Harriet.
   Ricky and David Nelson

4. These three English sisters of the 1800s were famous in literature. Their works, which include *Jane Eyre*, *Wuthering Heights*, and *Agnes Grey*, are still read by many today.
   Emily, Charlotte, and Anne Brontë

5. These brothers are credited with building the first successful airplane.
   Orville and Wilbur Wright

6. These four singing sisters were perhaps best known for their years on the *Lawrence Welk Show*.
   Lennon Sisters

7. These brothers from Biblical times are often thought to be the first two sons of Adam and Eve.
   Cain and Abel

8. These five comedian brothers often acted in vaudeville, movies, and, later, television.
   Marx Brothers—Harpo, Groucho, Zeppo, Chico, Gummo

9. These three sisters sang pop songs in the 1950s and '60s. They first appeared on *Arthur Godfry's Talent Scouts* in 1952. They went on to sign a very lucrative deal with Coca Cola and advertised with them for many years.
   McGuire Sisters

10. These two brothers are often thought of as the founders of Rome.
    Romulus and Remus

11. These two brothers formed a music and comedy team, giving live performances and starring in their own television shows in the latter part of the 20th century. They were famous for folk songs and for "arguing" with each other during performances.
    Smothers Brothers

12. These identical twin girls both changed their names and wrote advice columns in various newspapers for many, many years.
    Abigail Van Buren and Ann Landers

13. In the 1930s, these three sisters became the first female vocal group to earn a Gold Record. They recorded such popular hits as "Don't Sit Under the Apple Tree," "I'll Be With You in Apple Blossom Time," and the "Beer Barrel Polka." They sang many of their songs with Bing Crosby.
    Andrews Sisters

14. These two British acting sisters have both won Academy Awards. One sister won her first award for her role as Melanie in *Gone with the Wind* and the other for her role in Alfred Hitchcock's *Suspicion*.
    Olivia de Havilland and Joan Fontaine

15. These two brothers and two sisters are the children of Queen Elizabeth II and Prince Phillip.
    Prince Charles, Princess Anne, Princess Margaret, and Prince Edward

FACILITATOR: Ask participants for more facts about these famous siblings. What else do they know about them? Do they think one of the siblings is more famous than the other(s)? More talented? Which other siblings can they name that are famous? Do they have siblings themselves? If they were to become famous along with their sibling(s), what might it be for? Would they like to be famous?

First Ladies

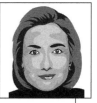

We usually think of first ladies as the wives of presidents. However, throughout history other women have also filled this position when the president was a bachelor or a widower or when his wife was simply unable to fulfill the required duties. There are many notable first ladies. The following first ladies are all wives of presidents and have all made their mark on the history of the United States. Can you name the husband of each first lady listed?

1. Abigail

2. Dolley

3. Thelma Catherine (Pat)

4. Claudia (Lady Bird)

5. Barbara

6. Betty

7. Martha

8. Hillary

9. Mamie

10. Bess

11. Anna Eleanor

12. Nancy

13. Mary Todd

14. Rosalynn

15. Jacqueline

16. Laura

17. Julia

18. Lou

First Ladies ANSWER SHEET

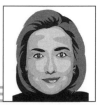

1. Abigail   **John Adams (also Leonard Filmore)**

2. Dolley   **James Madison**

3. Thelma Catherine (Pat)   **Richard Nixon**

4. Claudia (Lady Bird)   **Lyndon B. Johnson**

5. Barbara   **George H. W. Bush**

6. Betty   **Gerald Ford**

7. Martha   **George Washington (also Thomas Jefferson)**

8. Hillary   **Bill Clinton**

9. Mamie   **Dwight D. Eisenhower**

10. Bess   **Harry Truman**

11. Anna Eleanor   **Franklin D. Roosevelt (FDR)**

12. Nancy   **Ronald Reagan**

13. Mary Todd   **Abraham Lincoln**

14. Rosalynn   **Jimmy Carter**

15. Jacqueline   **John F. Kennedy (JFK)**

16. Laura   **George W. Bush**

17. Julia   **Ulysses S. Grant**

18. Lou   **Herbert Hoover**

FACILITATOR: *The American public has had a fascination with first ladies over the years. Ask participants why they think this is true. Who has been their favorite first lady? Which ones do they think have done the most for the country? What do they think the role of first lady should be? Have any overstepped their "boundaries"? If we have a female president, what do participants think her husband should be called? What should his role be? Should it be different than that of former first ladies? It would be helpful to have pictures of all the first ladies for this activity, including those not mentioned.*

Strengthen Your Mind, Volume Two by Einberger & Sellick. Copyright © 2008 by Health Professions Press, Inc.

Leaders in the World of Science and Nature

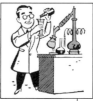

Science and nature go hand in hand. Many scientists are also naturalists. Many naturalists have a great interest in science. All are concerned with how things work and what the effects are on the environment. The following are descriptions of scientists and naturalists. Can you match the description on the left to the person on the right?

____ 1. This famous naturalist and author helped to preserve many sites, including Yosemite, and was the founder of the Sierra Club.

____ 2. This American naturalist was especially well known for identifying birds.

____ 3. An apple falling on his head helped this man explain the theory of gravity.

____ 4. This brilliant German-born physicist is best known for his theory of relativity.

____ 5. This American physician developed the first successful polio vaccine.

____ 6. This European physicist and chemist, along with her husband, was known for her work in the field of radioactivity.

____ 7. This president was known as a naturalist and conservationist and set aside during his presidency a great deal of land for national parks and wildlife areas.

____ 8. This English naturalist formed the modern evolutionary theory, including his belief in survival of the fittest.

____ 9. This English anthropologist is best known for her study of chimpanzees in Africa.

____ 10. This Polish astronomer was known as the Father of Modern Astronomy. He discovered that Earth rotates on its axis daily and travels around the sun yearly.

____ 11. This American marine biologist was also an author. She wrote *Silent Spring* and was an important figure in the modern environmental movement.

____ 12. This man proved that the planets revolve around the Sun, not Earth, as had been previously thought.

____ 13. This American scientist was also a politician. He invented the lightening rod and was best known for his work in the field of electricity.

____ 14. This modern politician and environmentalist has written and spoken a great deal about global warming.

____ 15. This scientist from the United States is known as the Father of Rocketry.

____ 16. This American physicist is known as the Father of the Atomic Bomb.

a. Copernicus

b. Albert Einstein

c. Marie Curie

d. Rachel Carson

e. Al Gore

f. Theodore Roosevelt

g. John J. Audubon

h. Charles Darwin

i. Jonas Salk

j. Jane Goodall

k. Galileo

l. Benjamin Franklin

m. Isaac Newton

n. Robert Oppenheimer

o. John Muir

p. Charles Goddard

Leaders in the World of Science and Nature
ANSWER SHEET

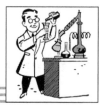

1. This famous naturalist and author helped to preserve many sites, including Yosemite, and was the founder of the Sierra Club.

o. John Muir

2. This American naturalist was especially well known for identifying birds.

g. John J. Audubon

3. An apple falling on his head helped this man explain the theory of gravity.

m. Isaac Newton

4. This brilliant German-born physicist is best known for his theory of relativity.

b. Albert Einstein

5. This American physician developed the first successful polio vaccine.

i. Jonas Salk

6. This European physicist and chemist, along with her husband, was known for her work in the field of radioactivity.

c. Marie Curie

7. This president was known as a naturalist and conservationist and set aside during his presidency a great deal of land for national parks and wildlife areas.

f. Theodore Roosevelt

8. This English naturalist formed the modern evolutionary theory, including his belief in survival of the fittest.

h. Charles Darwin

9. This English anthropologist is best known for her study of chimpanzees in Africa.

j. Jane Goodall

10. This Polish astronomer was known as the Father of Modern Astronomy. He discovered that Earth rotates on its axis daily and travels around the sun yearly.

a. Copernicus

11. This American marine biologist was also an author. She wrote *Silent Spring* and was an important figure in the modern environmental movement.

d. Rachel Carson

12. This man proved that the planets revolve around the Sun, not Earth, as had been previously thought.

k. Galileo

13. This American scientist was also a politician. He invented the lightening rod and was best known for his work in the field of electricity.

l. Benjamin Franklin

14. This modern politician and environmentalist has written and spoken a great deal about global warming.

e. Al Gore

15. This scientist from the United States is known as the Father of Rocketry.

p. Robert Goddard

16. This American physicist is known as the Father of the Atomic Bomb.

n. Robert Oppenheimer

FACILITATOR: *Many of these people will be well known to some, but some may not be. Discuss the different fields of science—physics, biology, environment, marine, chemistry, astronomy, and so forth. Which do participants like best? Did they take any of these subjects in school? Would they like to be a scientist? Which field would they choose? Can they name any other scientists or naturalists?*

 Strengthen Your Mind, Volume Two by Einberger & Sellick. Copyright © 2008 by Health Professions Press, Inc.

Military Leaders

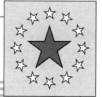

There have been many great military leaders during the past 3,000 years. Some have had a positive impact on their countries; others have had a negative one. All have made a difference in the history of the world. Can you name the following military leaders?

1. This man, who later went on to become the 18th U.S. president, was the lead Union General in the Civil War.

2. This World War II U.S. Army General was known as "Old Blood and Guts." He commanded forces mainly in North Africa, Sicily, France, and Germany.

3. This Confederate General was famous for his tactical brilliance and his nickname, which he received at Bull Run after refusing to retreat.

4. This Roman military and political leader had a profound impact on Roman civilization and the building of the Roman Empire. He was assassinated on the Ides of March (March 15).

5. This British Army Officer went on to become the Prime Minister of the United Kingdom in 1940 and one of the most influential leaders of the Allied forces.

6. This U.S. president led the Continental Army to victory in the American Revolutionary War in the late 1700s.

7. This revered Confederate General was the most celebrated of all officers during the Civil War. He was known for his victories against superior forces.

8. This German field marshal during WWII became known as "The Desert Fox" for his skill in leading troops in Northern Africa.

9. "In war, there is no substitute for victory," was the philosophy of this Army General who led troops in the Pacific during WWII.

10. This five-star general served as Supreme Commander of the Allied troops in Europe during WWII and later went on to become the 34th president of the United States.

11. This 15th-century French heroine fought against England to successfully recover her homeland, but she was later convicted of heresy and burned at the stake.

12. This Frenchman was a general during the French Revolution and later went on to become the Emperor of France in the early 1800s.

13. This man, General of the Armies, led the American Expeditionary Forces in WWI. His nickname was "Black Jack."

14. This U.S. General became chairman of the Joint Chiefs of Staff in 1989 and secretary of state under George W. Bush in 2001, the first African-American to hold that post.

Military Leaders ANSWER SHEET

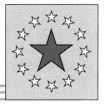

1. This man, who later went on to become the 18th U.S. president, was the lead Union General in the Civil War.
   Ulysses S. Grant

2. This World War II U.S. Army General was known as "Old Blood and Guts." He commanded forces mainly in North Africa, Sicily, France, and Germany.
   George S. Patton

3. This Confederate General was famous for his tactical brilliance and his nickname, which he received at Bull Run after refusing to retreat.
   Thomas "Stonewall" Jackson

4. This Roman military and political leader had a profound impact on Roman civilization and the building of the Roman Empire. He was assassinated on the Ides of March (March 15).
   Julius Caesar

5. This British Army Officer went on to become the Prime Minister of the United Kingdom in 1940 and one of the most influential leaders of the Allied forces.
   Winston Churchill

6. This U.S. president led the Continental Army to victory in the American Revolutionary War in the late 1700s.
   George Washington

7. This revered Confederate General was the most celebrated of all officers during the Civil War. He was known for his victories against superior forces.
   Robert E. Lee

8. This German field marshal during WWII became known as "The Desert Fox" for his skill in leading troops in Northern Africa.
   Erwin Rommel

9. "In war, there is no substitute for victory," was the philosophy of this Army General who led troops in the Pacific during WWII.
   Douglas MacArthur

10. This five-star general served as Supreme Commander of the Allied troops in Europe during WWII and later went on to become the 34th president of the United States.
    Dwight D. Eisenhower

11. This 15th-century French heroine fought against England to successfully recover her homeland, but she was later convicted of heresy and burned at the stake.
    Joan of Arc

12. This Frenchman was a general during the French Revolution and later went on to become the Emperor of France in the early 1800s.
    Napoleon Bonaparte

13. This man, General of the Armies, led the American Expeditionary Forces in WWI. His nickname was "Black Jack."
    John J. Pershing

14. This U.S. General became chairman of the Joint Chiefs of Staff in 1989 and secretary of state under George W. Bush in 2001, the first African-American to hold that post.
    Colin Powell

FACILITATOR: This is an especially significant activity for any participant who has served in one of the branches of the Armed Forces. Can they name the five branches? Which one did they serve in? What do they think of these leaders? Can they think of any others who had a significant impact on world history? How has the military changed over the years? How would it be different to be in military service today? Do they think that the draft should be re-instated? Should women serve alongside men in the service?

People and Characters Who Come in Threes

Sometimes three is better than one, whether in music, television, or comedy. These groups of people have achieved fame because of their act together. This worksheet will test your knowledge of people and characters who come in threes!

1. This trio is famously known as The Three Stooges.

2. This folk singing group from the 1960s had many popular hits, including "Lemon Tree."

3. This children's fairytale features these characters, who get chased by the farmer's wife.

4. This 1970s television comedy featured this trio, who lived together above their landlord Mr. Roper.

5. This rock band of the 1970s is known for the hits "Joy to the World" and "Mama Told Me Not to Come."

6. In the Bible, these men are known for bringing gifts to the baby Jesus.

7. In the popular television show *Bonanza*, these boys were the sons of main character Ben Cartwright.

8. In the early 1900s this trio of brothers entertained in vaudeville and comedy.

9. This Disney cartoon trio is the identical triplet nephews of Donald Duck.

10. This popular children's nursery rhyme featured these three men, all in a tub.

11. These three marketing characters are found on the boxes of Rice Krispies cereal.

12. In Christianity, it is said that God makes up these three beings, also called the trinity.

13. In the 1980s television show *Newhart*, these three characters were brothers who lived in the backwoods.

14. An expression that refers to the general public is "Every _____, _____, and _____."

15. In the 1950s and '60s, this folk and rock group was popular for many hits, including "Tom Dooley" and "Tijuana Jail."

16. This fictional music trio, which debuted in the 1950s, is made up of three chipmunks named . . .

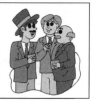

1. This trio is famously known as The Three Stooges.
   Larry, Moe, and Curly

2. This folk singing group from the 1960s had many popular hits, including "Lemon Tree."
   Peter, Paul, and Mary

3. This children's fairytale features these characters, who get chased by the farmer's wife.
   Three Blind Mice

4. This 1970s television comedy featured this trio, who lived together above their landlord Mr. Roper.
   Jack, Janet, and Chrissy

5. This rock band of the 1970s is known for the hits "Joy to the World" and "Mama Told Me Not to Come."
   Three Dog Night

6. In the Bible, these men are known for bringing gifts to the baby Jesus.
   Three Wise Men

7. In the popular television show *Bonanza*, these boys were the sons of main character Ben Cartwright.
   Adam, Hoss, and Little Joe

8. In the early 1900s this trio of brothers entertained in vaudeville and comedy.
   Groucho, Chico, and Harpo Marx

9. This Disney cartoon trio is the identical triplet nephews of Donald Duck.
   Huey, Dewey, and Louie

10. This popular children's nursery rhyme featured these three men, all in a tub.
    Butcher, Baker, and Candlestick Maker

11. These three marketing characters are found on the boxes of Rice Krispies cereal.
    Snap, Crackle, and Pop

12. In Christianity, it is said that God makes up these three beings, also called the trinity.
    Father, Son, and Holy Spirit

13. In the 1980s television show *Newhart*, these three characters were brothers who lived in the backwoods.
    Larry, Daryl, and Darryl

14. An expression that refers to the general public is "Every _____, _____, and _____."
    Tom, Dick, and Harry

15. In the 1950s and 1960s, this folk and rock group was popular for many hits, including "Tom Dooley" and "Tijuana Jail."
    The Kingston Trio

16. This fictional music trio, which debuted in the 1950s, is made up of three chipmunks named . . .
    Alvin, Simon, and Theodore

FACILITATOR: *If you can, bring in examples of the groups listed above (movie or television clips, cereal boxes, or music). Is everyone familiar with the groups of three and can anyone think of more groups of people who come in threes? How about things that come in threes? There a several terms that refer to groups of threes; can participants name some?*

People Known by Initials in Their Name

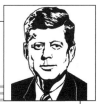

Some people reach a level of fame so great that they become known by their initials rather than by their full name. For some, initials are abbreviations of their full name. Regardless, there are many accomplished people both in politics and entertainment that are known by the initials in their name. Match the description of the person on the left with the initial or initials of the person on the right.

____ 1. This depression-era president is known for his New Deal legislation and modern day Social Security.

____ 2. This man is known for his poetry, most notably "The Waste Land," and was awarded the Nobel Prize in literature in 1948.

____ 3. This band, popular in the 1960s and early '70s, was best known for its hit song "Centerfold."

____ 4. This blues guitarist is widely known as "The King of Blues."

____ 5. This Irish novelist is well known for his series of children's books called *The Chronicles of Narnia*.

____ 6. This man is known for the creation of a chain of large retail department stores.

____ 7. This retired football player is best known for the highly publicized trial of the murder of his ex-wife.

____ 8. This psychologist is known for his work in behavior analysis and is famous for the creation of the operant conditioning chamber.

____ 9. This author and professor is best known for his books *The Lord of the Rings* and *The Hobbit*.

____ 10. This English writer is known for his novels *The War of the Worlds* and *The Island of Dr. Moreau*.

____ 11. This democratic president increased America's involvement in the Vietnam War and is known for designing Medicare and Medicaid.

____ 12. This Black Muslim Minister was known for his involvement in politics and was assassinated at the age 39.

____ 13. This confederate general is known for his many victories during the Civil War.

____ 14. This novelist of the Jazz Age is known for many works, among them *The Great Gatsby*.

____ 15. The nation was shocked when this well-liked democratic president was assassinated in 1963.

a. CS Lewis

b. LBJ

c. JC Penney

d. OJ Simpson

e. FDR

f. Robert E Lee

g. TS Eliot

h. BB King

i. F Scott Fitzgerald

j. JRR Tolkien

k. JFK

l. J Geils Band

m. BF Skinner

n. HG Wells

o. Malcolm X

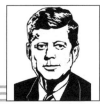

1. This depression-era president is known for his New Deal legislation and modern day Social Security.

    e. FDR

2. This man is known for his poetry, most notably "The Waste Land," and was awarded the Nobel Prize in literature in 1948.

    g. TS Eliot

3. This band, popular in the 1960s and early '70s, was best known for its hit song "Centerfold."

    l. J Geils Band

4. This blues guitarist is widely known as "The King of Blues."

    h. BB King

5. This Irish novelist is well known for his series of children's books called *The Chronicles of Narnia*.

    a. CS Lewis

6. This man is known for the creation of a chain of large retail department stores.

    c. JC Penney

7. This retired football player is best known for the highly publicized trial of the murder of his ex-wife.

    d. OJ Simpson

8. This psychologist is known for his work in behavior analysis and is famous for the creation of the operant conditioning chamber.

    m. BF Skinner

9. This author and professor is best known for his books *The Lord of the Rings* and *The Hobbit*.

    j. JRR Tolkien

10. This English writer is known for his novels *The War of the Worlds* and *The Island of Dr. Moreau*.

    n. HG Wells

11. This democratic president increased America's involvement in the Vietnam War and is known for designing Medicare and Medicaid.

    b. LBJ

12. This Black Muslim Minister was known for his involvement in politics and was assassinated at the age 39.

    o. Malcolm X

13. This confederate general is known for his many victories during the Civil War.

    f. Robert E Lee

14. This novelist of the Jazz Age is known for many works, among them *The Great Gatsby*.

    i. F Scott Fitzgerald

15. The nation was shocked when this well-liked democratic president was assassinated in 1963.

    k. JFK

FACILITATOR: *This is only a partial list of people known by their initials. Use this worksheet as a discussion point for the following questions: Do you have any friends or family who are called by their initials? How do you think these "nick-names" come about? Outside of initials, can you think of people who are famous for their middle name?*

People with Food Products Named After Them

Some inventors are so proud of their product that they put their name on it. Others name their invention after a beloved family member or friend. Below are descriptions of products and people on the left and a list of products and people on the right. Match the product with the person.

____ 1. This man is considered the founder of the frozen food industry, but his name is most commonly found on bags of frozen vegetables.

____ 2. The creativity and baking skills of this woman led to the development of these delicious cookies, which can be found in malls across America.

____ 3. This man had a passion for popcorn and his brand continues to be one of the most popular today.

____ 4. Delicious, high-quality chocolate candies are named after this woman and her son, who started the company the candies are named after in 1921.

____ 5. This nonalcoholic drink is made from ginger ale, grenadine, and orange juice and is named after one of the most well-known child stars.

____ 6. This small, cylindrical chocolate candy has been around for over 100 years and was named after the inventor's daughter.

____ 7. This popular drink was created in Texas in 1885, and it is generally believed that the product is named after this doctor.

____ 8. This man advocated for healthy eating habits in the 1800s and is known for the creation of graham flour, which led to the development of the graham cracker, still popular in stores today.

____ 9. These delicious chocolates are named for a legendary English woman who is known for riding her horse through town, naked, to protest the high rate of taxes for the residents.

____ 10. This corporation, which traces its history back to 1930, produces baked goods worldwide. It is especially known for its bread and is named after the founder's daughter.

____ 11. This Vermont-based ice cream company is named after two best friends who created the company as well as many of the exotic flavors that it sells.

____ 12. Many believe that this candy bar was named after a famous baseball player; however, others contend that it was named after President Grover Cleveland's daughter.

____ 13. This company is named after its founder and is best known for its corn flakes cereal.

____ 14. This type of tea is named after a British prime minister who received the tea as a gift in the 1830s.

____ 15. This company is known for its salad dressing and is named for its founder, a person who donates 100% of the company's proceeds to charity.

a. Tootsie Roll

b. See's Candy

c. Dr. Pepper

d. Sylvester Graham

e. Earl Grey

f. Kellogg's

g. Clarence Birdseye

h. Debbi Fields

i. Orville Redenbacher

j. Ben and Jerry's

k. Newman's Own

l. Godiva

m. Shirley Temple

n. Sara Lee

o. Baby Ruth

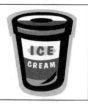

People with Food Products Named After Them ANSWER SHEET

1. This man is considered the founder of the frozen food industry, but his name is most commonly found on bags of frozen vegetables.

    g. Clarence Birdseye

2. The creativity and baking skills of this woman led to the development of these delicious cookies, which can be found in malls across America.

    h. Debbi Fields

3. This man had a passion for popcorn and his brand continues to be one of the most popular today.

    i. Orville Redenbacher

4. Delicious, high-quality chocolate candies are named after this woman and her son, who started the company the candies are named after in 1921.

    b. See's Candy

5. This nonalcoholic drink is made from ginger ale, grenadine, and orange juice and is named after one of the most well-known child stars.

    m. Shirley Temple

6. This small, cylindrical chocolate candy has been around for over 100 years and was named after the inventor's daughter.

    a. Tootsie Roll

7. This popular drink was created in Texas in 1885, and it is generally believed that the product is named after this doctor.

    c. Dr. Pepper

8. This man advocated for healthy eating habits in the 1800s and is known for the creation of graham flour, which led to the development of the graham cracker, still popular in stores today.

    d. Sylvester Graham

9. These delicious chocolates are named for a legendary English woman who is known for riding her horse through town, naked, to protest the high rate of taxes for the residents.

    l. Godiva

10. This corporation, which traces its history back to 1930, produces baked goods worldwide. It is especially known for its bread and is named after the founder's daughter.

    n. Sara Lee

11. This Vermont-based ice cream company is named after two best friends who created the company as well as many of the exotic flavors that it sells.

    j. Ben and Jerry's

12. Many believe that this candy bar was named after a famous baseball player; however, others contend that it was named after President Grover Cleveland's daughter.

    o. Baby Ruth

13. This company is named after its founder and is best known for its corn flakes cereal.

    f. Kellogg's

14. This type of tea is named after a British prime minister who received the tea as a gift in the 1830s.

    e. Earl Grey

15. This company is known for its salad dressing and is named for its founder, a person who donates 100% of the company's proceeds to charity.

    k. Newman's Own

FACILITATOR: *Bring in a sample of some or all of these products so that people can try them. Has everyone had each of the products? If you were to name a product after someone, who would it be? What would the product be? Can you think of any other food products that are named after people who are not on this list? Would you change the name of any of these products to something that would be a better fit?*

Places and Things Named for People

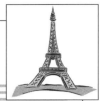

Not only do people name products after other people, but places and things are often namesakes as well. Some of the most noted tourist destinations in the world have been named for people, including our own continent. Match the description on the left to the answer on the right.

____ 1. Many contend that these two continents were named after Italian explorer Amerigo Vespucci, who believed that the continents were a previously undiscovered world.

____ 2. This Chicago baseball park is named after its owner, the same person who owns one of the most famous chewing gum companies in the world.

____ 3. This famous French landmark, named after its designer, stands 990 feet tall and was built for the 1889 International Exposition.

____ 4. This Los Angeles destination, originally called Mann's Chinese Theater, is the home of nearly 200 celebrity handprints, footprints, and autographs.

____ 5. This famous comet that was last seen in 1986 is visible every 75 to 76 years and was named after an English astronomer.

____ 6. This performing arts center in Washington, DC, was designated as a memorial to a famous president who was assassinated in 1963.

____ 7. This theme park is known for being the "Happiest Place on Earth" and is named after its creator, a legend in animation.

____ 8. This nationwide financial services company has over 6,000 branches and is named after the two men who created it in 1852.

____ 9. As one of the largest auto companies in the United States, this company was named after its founder and is over 100 years old.

____ 10. Over ten towers and plazas throughout the world are named after this real estate mogul and entertainer, one of the richest men in the United States.

____ 11. This item, popular with young children, was named after Theodore Roosevelt.

____ 12. Named after its creator, this line of foot care products includes shoes, inserts, lotions, and other foot-pampering items.

____ 13. Located in Vatican City, this site is named after one of the 12 apostles of Jesus.

____ 14. This Polish-born woman created a beauty empire and created a cosmetics business named after herself.

a. Wells Fargo

b. Eiffel Tower

c. Helena Rubenstein

d. Halley's Comet

e. Donald Trump

f. Dr. Scholl's

g. Grauman's Chinese Theatre

h. North and South America

i. St. Peter's Basilica

j. Disneyland

k. Ford Motor Company

l. The Kennedy Center

m. Teddy Bear

n. Wrigley Field

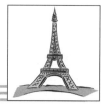

1. Many contend that these two continents were named after Italian explorer Amerigo Vespucci, who believed that the continents were a previously undiscovered world.

    h. North and South America

2. This Chicago baseball park is named after its owner, the same person who owns one of the most famous chewing gum companies in the world.

    n. Wrigley Field

3. This famous French landmark, named after its designer, stands 990 feet tall and was built for the 1889 International Exposition.

    b. Eiffel Tower

4. This Los Angeles destination, originally called Mann's Chinese Theater, is the home of nearly 200 celebrity handprints, footprints, and autographs.

    g. Grauman's Chinese Theatre

5. This famous comet that was last seen in 1986 is visible every 75 to 76 years and was named after an English astronomer.

    d. Halley's Comet

6. This performing arts center in Washington, DC, was designated as a memorial to a famous president who was assassinated in 1963.

    l. The Kennedy Center

7. This theme park is known for being the "Happiest Place on Earth" and is named after its creator, a legend in animation.

    j. Disneyland

8. This nationwide financial services company has over 6,000 branches and is named after the two men who created it in 1852.

    a. Wells Fargo

9. As one of the largest auto companies in the United States, this company was named after its founder and is over 100 years old.

    k. Ford Motor Company

10. Over ten towers and plazas throughout the world are named after this real estate mogul and entertainer, one of the richest men in the United States.

    e. Donald Trump

11. This item, popular with young children, was named after Theodore Roosevelt.

    m. Teddy Bear

12. Named after its creator, this line of foot care products includes shoes, inserts, lotions, and other foot-pampering items.

    f. Dr. Scholl's

13. Located in Vatican City, this site is named after one of the 12 apostles of Jesus.

    i. St. Peter's Basilica

14. This Polish-born woman created a beauty empire and created a cosmetics business named after herself.

    c. Helena Rubenstein

FACILITATOR: *These well-known products and places are named after people. Many of your participants have probably used them or traveled to these sites at some time. Ask the group if they are familiar with each of these. Has anyone used any of the items? Has anyone traveled to any of the locations listed above? Why do participants think these places and things were named as they were? What other places and things are named after people? What qualities should a person have in order to have something named after him or her? If you were to create a product, whom would you name it after and why? How about a place? Has anything or a person ever been named after you?*

Popular Song Titles that Contain a Person's Name

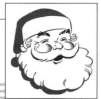

Songs are often named for a particular person. Sometimes this person may be someone known to the writer, and other times the name may just fit the song. The following descriptions are of common song titles that contain the first name of a person. Can you name the person?

1. "Bring back, bring back" begins the chorus of this Scottish song.

2. This 1911 Irving Berlin song refers to a specific "band."

3. "The pipes are calling" in this English song, sung to the Irish tune of "Londonderry Air."

4. This 1964 song from a movie of the same name was popularized by Carol Channing in the movie and later by Louis Armstrong.

5. This 1960s country song refers to a man from a town in Oklahoma. It was made famous by Merle Haggard.

6. This song from the late 1800s is about a miner 49'er and a woman with size 9 shoes.

7. This "old sweet song" is now the state song of a southeastern coastal state and was a hallmark of Ray Charles in the 1960s.

8. This 1917 hit, most famously recorded by the Andrew Sisters in the 1940s, asks "Please tell me dear, what makes me love you so? / You're not handsome, it's true / But when I look at you . . . "

9. "She's the sweetest little rose this garden ever grew" is a lyric included in this popular song from 1896.

10. "Oh, oh, oh, what a gal" this female is, the title song in an Eddie Cantor movie of the same name.

11. This Christmas song was first sung on Eddie Cantor's radio show in 1934. "You better watch out, you better not cry" the song warns.

12. "I'll do the cooking darling, I'll pay the rent / I know I've done you wrong" goes the chorus of this song from 1902, often sung by Louis Armstrong.

13. This barbershop classic from the early 1900s is also a name of an international organization of women's barbershop harmony.

14. Though this popular song was written in 1921, it was used later in Truman's presidential campaign. It was perfect in that it had his first name as part of the title!

15. "Days are never blue / After all is said and done, there is really only one / Oh,_____,_____, it's you!" are lyrics in this early 1900s love song about a woman.

Popular Song Titles that Contain a Person's Name
ANSWER SHEET

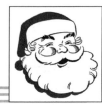

1. "Bring back, bring back" begins the chorus of this Scottish song.
   "My Bonnie Lies Over the Ocean"
2. This 1911 Irving Berlin song refers to a specific "band."
   "Alexander's Ragtime Band"
3. "The pipes are calling" in this English song, sung to the Irish tune of "Londonderry Air."
   "Danny Boy"
4. This 1964 song from a movie of the same name was popularized by Carol Channing in the movie and later by Louis Armstrong.
   "Hello Dolly"
5. This 1960s country song refers to a man from a town in Oklahoma. It was made famous by Merle Haggard.
   "Okie from Muskogee"
6. This song from the late 1800s is about a miner 49'er and a woman with size 9 shoes.
   "Oh My Darling, Clementine"
7. This "old sweet song" is now the state song of a southeastern coastal state and was a hallmark of Ray Charles in the 1960s.
   "Georgia on My Mind"
8. This 1917 hit, most famously recorded by the Andrew Sisters in the 1940s, asks "Please tell me dear, what makes me love you so? / You're not handsome, it's true / But when I look at you . . . "
   "Oh, Johnny, Oh Johnny, Oh!"
9. "She's the sweetest little rose this garden ever grew" is a lyric included in this popular song from 1896.
   "Sweet Rosie O'Grady"
10. "Oh, oh, oh, what a gal" this female is, the title song in an Eddie Cantor movie of the same name.
    "If You Knew Susie"
11. This Christmas song was first sung on Eddie Cantor's radio show in 1934. "You better watch out, you better not cry" the song warns.
    "Santa Claus Is Coming to Town"
12. "I'll do the cooking darling, I'll pay the rent / I know I've done you wrong" goes the chorus of this song from 1902, often sung by Louis Armstrong.
    "Won't You Come Home, Bill Bailey?"
13. This barbershop classic from the early 1900s is also a name of an international organization of women's barbershop harmony.
    "Sweet Adeline"
14. Though this popular song was written in 1921, it was used later in Truman's presidential campaign. It was perfect in that it had his first name as part of the title!
    "I'm Just Wild About Harry"
15. "Days are never blue / After all is said and done, there is really only one / Oh,_____, _____, it's you!" are lyrics in this early 1900s love song about a woman.
    "Margie"

FACILITATOR: *Like all activities having to do with music, it would be great to have some of the lyrics for these songs printed out and/or have some of the recordings. Which of these songs have participants sung? Which other songs have a person's name in the title? For example, "My Heart Belongs to Daddy," "Mack the Knife," "Ida Sweet as Apple Cider," and so forth.*

Presidential Facts

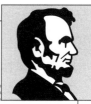

We have had 43 presidents since our democracy began in 1776. Much has been written about each president, some good, some bad. The following facts each pertain to one president specifically. Many of these facts are relatively unknown and are not meant to be answered correctly, but are just meant for fun! Can you guess who any of these presidents are?

1. Which president was so large that he got stuck in a bathtub?

2. Which president was the first to wear a beard while in office?

3. Who was the oldest president in office?

4. Who was the only president to refuse to eat broccoli?

5. Which president served the longest?

6. Whose library of approximately 6,000 books became the basis for the Library of Congress?

7. Which president was the first to visit China while in office?

8. Which president was arrested for driving his horse too fast?

9. Who was the only Roman Catholic president?

10. Who was the first president to ride to his inauguration in a car?

11. Which president was a managing general partner of the Texas Rangers?

12. Who was the first president elected who lived west of the Mississippi?

13. Who was the first president to give a speech on television?

14. Which president was the first to ride in an airplane?

15. Which four presidents were assassinated?

16. Who was the only president to earn a doctorate?

17. Who was the only president to have been a Rhodes Scholar?

18. Which president was the smallest?

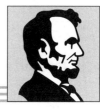

Presidential Facts ANSWER SHEET

1. Which president was so large that he got stuck in a bathtub?
    William Taft—so a new one was installed that could hold four grown men!

2. Which president was the first to wear a beard while in office?
    Abraham Lincoln

3. Who was the oldest president in office?
    Ronald Reagan, who was age 69 upon entering and 77 upon leaving

4. Who was the only president to refuse to eat broccoli?
    George H. W. Bush

5. Which president served the longest?
    Franklin D. Roosevelt (FDR), who served three terms and part of his fourth

6. Whose library of approximately 6,000 books became the basis for the Library of Congress?
    Thomas Jefferson

7. Which president was the first to visit China while in office?
    Richard Nixon

8. Which president was arrested for driving his horse too fast?
    Ulysses S. Grant, who was fined $20

9. Who was the only Roman Catholic president?
    John F. Kennedy (JFK)

10. Who was the first president to ride to his inauguration in a car?
    Warren G. Harding

11. Which president was a managing general partner of the Texas Rangers?
    George W. Bush

12. Who was the first president elected who lived west of the Mississippi?
    Herbert Hoover

13. Who was the first president to give a speech on television?
    Harry S. Truman

14. Which president was the first to ride in an airplane?
    Theodore ("Teddy") Roosevelt, who flew for 4 minutes in a plane built by the Wright brothers in 1910

15. Which four presidents were assassinated?
    Abraham Lincoln, James A. Garfield, William McKinley, and John F. Kennedy

16. Who was the only president to earn a doctorate?
    Woodrow Wilson, although he could not read until he was 9 years old

17. Who was the only president to have been a Rhodes Scholar?
    Bill Clinton

18. Which president was the smallest?
    James Madison, who was 5'4" tall, 100 pounds

FACILITATOR: Once completed, ask participants for other interesting facts they know regarding presidents. How many presidents can they name? Who do they think was the best president? Why? Who was the worst? What do they think of the current president? Should a president now be limited to two terms? When did they first vote? For whom?

Strengthen Your Mind, Volume Two by Einberger & Sellick. Copyright © 2008 by Health Professions Press, Inc.

Terms for Groups of People

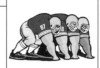

Whether small or large, groups of people gather for all reasons: educational, social, political, or just for fun. Most people have belonged to at least one type of group at some point in their lives, as it is human nature to want to be a part of something. For this worksheet, read the description of a type of group on the left and find the name of the group on the right.

____ 1. A group of people who gather for a specific purpose, often religious, is called a what?

____ 2. A term for a group of teenagers who sometimes exclude others.

____ 3. A secretive group of people who subscribe to a specific belief or purpose, often with a negative connotation.

____ 4. A group of people who play sports together.

____ 5. A term for a group of young people who band together and often perform illegal activities.

____ 6. A group of people within a larger group.

____ 7. A group of people known for their trade or craft.

____ 8. People who follow a certain political belief are said to belong to a what?

____ 9. A group of people called together to capture a criminal.

____ 10. An organization of workers who bargain with an employer.

____ 11. A group of military people, sometimes called soldiers.

____ 12. A term for a group of people who are alike in age, education, or other quality.

____ 13. A group temporarily gathered together for a given project or activity.

____ 14. An association of people who have a common goal or interest and who normally pay dues.

____ 15. A large number of people gathered into a space.

____ 16. A group of people involved in operating a ship is sometimes called a what?

____ 17. A portion of a group of people compromised of more than one half of the group.

____ 18. A small group of people gathered to answer questions from others or to discuss an issue.

a. cult

b. task force

c. troop

d. clique

e. guild

f. union

g. panel

h. crew

i. congregation

j. peer group

k. majority

l. crowd

m. party

n. gang

o. posse

p. club

q. faction

r. team

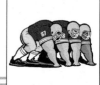

1. A group of people who gather for a specific purpose, often religious, is called a what? — **i. congregation**

2. A term for a group of teenagers who sometimes exclude others. — **d. clique**

3. A secretive group of people who subscribe to a specific belief or purpose, often with a negative connotation. — **a. cult**

4. A group of people who play sports together. — **r. team**

5. A term for a group of young people who band together and often perform illegal activities. — **n. gang**

6. A group of people within a larger group. — **q. faction**

7. A group of people known for their trade or craft. — **e. guild**

8. People who follow a certain political belief are said to belong to a what? — **m. party**

9. A group of people called together to capture a criminal. — **o. posse**

10. An organization of workers who bargain with an employer. — **f. union**

11. A group of military people, sometimes called soldiers. — **c. troop**

12. A term for a group of people who are alike in age, education, or other quality. — **j. peer group**

13. A group temporarily gathered together for a given project or activity. — **b. task force**

14. An association of people who have a common goal or interest and who normally pay dues. — **p. club**

15. A large number of people gathered into a space. — **l. crowd**

16. A group of people involved in operating a ship is sometimes called a what? — **h. crew**

17. A portion of a group of people compromised of more than one half of the group. — **k. majority**

18. A small group of people gathered to answer questions from others or to discuss an issue. — **g. panel**

FACILITATOR: *This is a good worksheet to bring up a discussion about types of groups that individuals have belonged to. What types of clubs or organizations have participants belonged to as a child? A teenager? An adult? A retiree? Are there any clubs or groups that you wanted to join, but never did? Do you have a favorite club? There are many more words that describe groups. Compile an A–Z list of these words for an additional activity.*

*T*ime Magazine Person of the Year

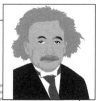

Time Magazine, the first weekly news magazine, was first published in 1923. Its editors selected their first "Person of the Year" in 1927. People have been chosen for the impact that they have had in the world, whether good or bad. The following people have each been selected at least one time over nearly 100 years. Can you name them?

1. 1927—This man's solo flight across the Atlantic Ocean put him on the cover. He is the first and youngest person to have ever been chosen.

2. 1932, 1934, and 1941—This man, the only one to have been selected three times, was first chosen as he became president and brought with him the "New Deal."

3. 1936—King Edward VIII of England abdicated the throne in order to marry this woman, the first woman to be named "Person of the Year."

4. 1938—This man was probably the most controversial of all of *Time*'s choices. In this year, he became "the greatest threatening force that the democratic, freedom-loving world faces today."

5. 1940, 1949 (Man of the Half Century)—In his first statement to the House of Commons, this Prime Minister declared, "I have nothing to offer but blood, tears, toils, and sweat."

6. 1945, 1948—This person's tough decision to order an atomic bomb be dropped on Hiroshima made him man of the year in 1945. In 1948, it was his resolve and ability to beat Thomas E. Dewey for the presidency.

7. 1952—The British people, upon the coronation of this young woman, hoped that she, like Queen Victoria in the past, would be a sign of a great future for the Commonwealth.

8. 1958—This popular French leader turned France around late in the 1950s, "giving France back their pride for the first time since early in WWII."

9. 1963—This man was the leader of the Southern Christian Leadership Conference and spent his all-too-short life preaching nonviolence.

10. 1989 & Man of the Decade—This Russian leader changed the face of the Soviet empire and thereby changed its relationship with the rest of the world, making possible the end of the cold war.

11. 1994—This Catholic leader set forth his vision of morality and urged the world to follow it.

12. 2001—This man, the mayor of New York City during the bombing of the Twin Towers, worked tirelessly to hold the city together in the midst of crisis.

13. 2005—This husband and wife Microsoft billionaires and a rock star were selected as Good Samaritans. All have the goal to stamp out world hunger.

14. Person of the 20th Century—This scientist was described as the genius among geniuses, one who discovered, merely by thinking about it, that the universe was not as it seemed.

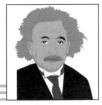

1. 1927—This man's solo flight across the Atlantic Ocean put him on the cover. He is the first and youngest person to have ever been chosen.
   Charles Lindbergh
2. 1932, 1934, and 1941—This man, the only one to have been selected three times, was first chosen as he became president and brought with him the "New Deal."
   Franklin D. Roosevelt
3. 1936—King Edward VIII of England abdicated the throne in order to marry this woman, the first woman to be named "Person of the Year."
   Wallis Warfield Simpson
4. 1938—This man was probably the most controversial of all of *Time*'s choices. In this year, he became "the greatest threatening force that the democratic, freedom-loving world faces today."
   Adolph Hitler
5. 1940, 1949 (Man of the Half Century)—In his first statement to the House of Commons, this Prime Minister declared, "I have nothing to offer but blood, tears, toils, and sweat."
   Winston Churchill
6. 1945, 1948—This person's tough decision to order an atomic bomb be dropped on Hiroshima made him man of the year in 1945. In 1948, it was his resolve and ability to beat Thomas E. Dewey for the presidency.
   Harry S. Truman
7. 1952—The British people, upon the coronation of this young woman, hoped that she, like Queen Victoria in the past, would be a sign of a great future for the Commonwealth
   Queen Elizabeth II
8. 1958—This popular French leader turned France around late in the 1950s, "giving France back their pride for the first time since early in WWII."
   Charles de Gaulle
9. 1963—This man was the leader of the Southern Christian Leadership Conference and spent his all-too-short life preaching nonviolence.
   Martin Luther King Jr.
10. 1989 & Man of the Decade—This Russian leader changed the face of the Soviet empire and thereby changed its relationship with the rest of the world, making possible the end of the cold war.
    Mikhail Gorbachev
11. 1994—This Catholic leader set forth his vision of morality and urged the world to follow it.
    Pope John Paul II
12. 2001—This man, the mayor of New York City during the bombing of the World Trade Center, worked tirelessly to hold the city together in the midst of crisis.
    Rudolph Giuliani
13. 2005—This husband and wife Microsoft billionaires and a rock star were selected as Good Samaritans. All have the goal to stamp out world hunger.
    Bill Gates, Melinda Gates, and Bono
14. Person of the 20th Century—This scientist was described as the genius among geniuses, one who discovered, merely by thinking about it, that the universe was not as it seemed.
    Albert Einstein

FACILITATOR: These people are certainly among the most memorable in history. What do participants know about them? Do they believe that they indeed did have a profound impact on the world? What about Hitler? Should Time have chosen a person such as this? If the participants could be on any magazine cover, what would it be and for what reason? If they could change the future of the world, how would they do it?

Television Hosts

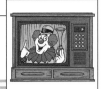

Quiz shows have been around since the early days of television. The first was *Pantomime Quiz*, which premiered in 1948. In the 1950s, many quiz shows jumped on the bandwagon. Contestants were put in an isolation booth, awaiting their turn to answer questions. Late in the 1950s, a scandal rocked the industry when it was discovered that certain contestants had been given answers ahead of time. Although this scandal had a negative impact on most viewers, quiz shows have survived and, in fact, are very popular today. Can you match the people on the left to the quiz shows they hosted on the right?

___ 1. Hugh Downs

___ 2. John Daly

___ 3. Groucho Marx

___ 4. Dick Clark

___ 5. Ralph Edwards

___ 6. Bill Cullen

___ 7. Pat Sajak (and sidekick Vanna White)

___ 8. Gary Moore

___ 9. Monty Hall

___ 10. Alex Trebek

___ 11. Johnny Carson

___ 12. Gene Rayburn

___ 13. Allen Ludden

___ 14. Peter Marshall

___ 15. Wink Martindale

___ 16. Richard Dawson

___ 17. Bert Parks

___ 18. Jack Barry

a. *You Bet Your Life*

b. *The Price Is Right*

c. *Let's Make a Deal*

d. *Match Game*

e. *Break the Bank*

f. *What's My Line?*

g. *Jeopardy*

h. *Truth or Consequences*

i. *Hollywood Squares*

j. *Family Feud*

k. *Who Do You Trust?*

l. *Twenty-One*

m. *The $10,000 Pyramid*

n. *Tic-Tac-Dough*

o. *I've Got a Secret*

p. *Password*

q. *Wheel of Fortune*

r. *Concentration*

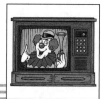

1.	Hugh Downs	r.	*Concentration*
2.	John Daly	f.	*What's My Line?*
3.	Groucho Marx	a.	*You Bet Your Life*
4.	Dick Clark	m.	*The $10,000 Pyramid*
5.	Ralph Edwards	h.	*Truth or Consequences*
6.	Bill Cullen	b.	*The Price Is Right*
7.	Pat Sajak (and sidekick Vanna White)	q.	*Wheel of Fortune*
8.	Gary Moore	o.	*I've Got a Secret*
9.	Monty Hall	c.	*Let's Make a Deal*
10.	Alex Trebek	g.	*Jeopardy*
11.	Johnny Carson	k.	*Who Do You Trust?*
12.	Gene Rayburn	d.	*Match Game*
13.	Allen Ludden	p.	*Password*
14.	Peter Marshall	i.	*Hollywood Squares*
15.	Wink Martindale	n.	*Tic-Tac-Dough*
16.	Richard Dawson	j.	*Family Feud*
17.	Bert Parks	e.	*Break the Bank*
18.	Jack Barry	l.	*Twenty-One*

FACILITATOR: *Quiz show history is long and interesting. Ask each participant which is his or her favorite? Which others do they remember? Did they listen to quiz shows on the radio, such as* Information, Please *and* Stop the Music? *Do they remember the 1950s scandal of television quiz shows? Do they think today's quiz shows are honest? Why is it that almost all quiz show hosts are male? How many watch* Jeopardy *and/or* Wheel of Fortune *today? You could engage participants in a quiz show following this activity, based on the rules of one of their favorite shows. Possibilities may be* Jeopardy, The Price Is Right, *or* What's My Line?

Who Invented What?

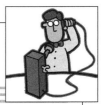

Things have been invented for thousands of years. Many of the earliest "inventors" were not even aware that they were inventing anything! In the last few hundred years, though, patents have been awarded to inventors to protect their inventions. Can you match each invention on the left with its inventor on the right?

____ 1. Mass production of the automobile in the early 1900s

____ 2. Light bulb in the 1870s

____ 3. Bifocals in the 1760s

____ 4. Frozen food in 1924

____ 5. Laws of motion in 1687

____ 6. The cotton gin in 1793

____ 7. An innovative printing press machine that used movable type c. 1450

____ 8. The theory of relativity beginning in 1907

____ 9. The first successful polio vaccine in 1955

____ 10. The telephone in 1876; he made the first transcontinental phone call from New York City in 1915 to Thomas Watson in San Francisco.

____ 11. In 1821, this young blind man devised a system of reading and writing for blind people.

____ 12. In 1846, he made the first functional sewing machine.

____ 13. Mechanical reaper in 1834

____ 14. Electrical telegraph in 1837

____ 15. Peanut butter

____ 16. The "roll film" camera in 1888 and the Kodak Company

____ 17. In 1807, he built the first commercial steamboat, which carried passengers between New York City and Albany, NY.

____ 18. The process of pasteurization in the 1860s

a. Louis Braille

b. Eli Whitney

c. Henry Ford

d. Louis Pasteur

e. George Washington Carver

f. Albert Einstein

g. Thomas Edison

h. Alexander Graham Bell

i. Robert Fulton

j. Sir Isaac Newton

k. Benjamin Franklin

l. Cyrus McCormick

m. George Eastman

n. Johannes Gutenberg

o. Samuel Morse

p. Jonas Salk

q. Clarence Birdseye

r. Elias Howe

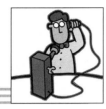

Who Invented What? ANSWER SHEET

1.	Mass production of the automobile in the early 1900s	c.	**Henry Ford**
2.	Light bulb in the 1870s	g.	**Thomas Edison**
3.	Bifocals in the 1760s	k.	**Benjamin Franklin**
4.	Frozen food in 1924	q.	**Clarence Birdseye**
5.	Laws of motion in 1687	j.	**Sir Isaac Newton**
6.	The cotton gin in 1793	b.	**Eli Whitney**
7.	An innovative printing press machine that used movable type c. 1450	n.	**Johannes Gutenberg**
8.	The theory of relativity beginning in 1907	f.	**Albert Einstein**
9.	The first successful polio vaccine in 1955	p.	**Jonas Salk**
10.	The telephone in 1876; he made the first transcontinental phone call from New York City in 1915 to Thomas Watson in San Francisco.	h.	**Alexander Graham Bell**
11.	In 1821, this young blind man devised a system of reading and writing for blind people.	a.	**Louis Braille**
12.	In 1846, he made the first functional sewing machine.	r.	**Elias Howe**
13.	Mechanical reaper in 1834	l.	**Cyrus McCormick**
14.	Electrical telegraph in 1837	o.	**Samuel Morse**
15.	Peanut butter	e.	**George Washington Carver**
16.	The "roll film" camera in 1888 and the Kodak Company	m.	**George Eastman**
17.	In 1807, he built the first commercial steamboat, which carried passengers between New York City and Albany, NY.	i.	**Robert Fulton**
18.	The process of pasteurization in the 1860s	d.	**Louis Pasteur**

FACILITATOR: *This is a great subject to tap into the creative side of participants. Ask which inventions have changed their lives the most. Which are most important to society? Can they think of things that have been invented/ produced that seem to make no sense—like the pet rock? Is there something that they would like to invent? Have they ever thought about trying to follow through on creating an invention? Have they ever known anyone who invented anything?*

Who Wrote What?

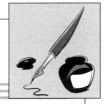

People have written books for thousands of years. Many of these books have withstood the passage of time. Others were important only to the writers themselves. Can you name the following writers who have written books that are considered classics in world literature?

___ 1. This man wrote books of life on the Mississippi River. Huck Finn and Tom Sawyer were two of his favorite characters.

___ 2. This French author was one of the first to write science fiction. His most famous works include *Around the World in 80 Days* and *Twenty Thousand Leagues Under the Sea.*

___ 3. This man lived in ancient Greece and was credited for writing a series of fables that all had a moral lesson.

___ 4. This Englishman was famous for many books, some of which were made into movies that did equally well. His books include *David Copperfield, A Christmas Carol,* and *The Adventures of Oliver Twist.*

___ 5. This American writer was best known for her book *Little Women,* a novel based on her life growing up with three sisters.

___ 6. This American writer and educator's name is often thought of as synonymous with the dictionary.

___ 7. This author received a Pulitzer Prize in 1953 for *The Old Man and the Sea.* Though he had a troubled personal life, he received great acclaim for other books, including *The Sun Also Rises, A Farewell to Arms,* and *For Whom the Bell Tolls.*

___ 8. One of the best-known American authors of the 20th century, this man from Salinas, CA, wrote many books about that area, including *Cannery Row.* Other books include *The Grapes of Wrath* and *Of Mice and Men.*

___ 9. This Danish author was best known for writing fairy tales, including *The Ugly Duckling, The Emperor's New Clothes,* and *The Little Mermaid.*

___ 10. This English author, nicknamed "The Bard of Avon," wrote dozens of plays, sonnets, and poems. Some of his most famous include *Macbeth, Hamlet,* and *Romeo and Juliet.*

___ 11. This 20th-century American author spent much of her life in China. Her most famous book is *The Good Earth.*

___ 12. This 19th-century poet was thought by many to be America's best poet, though his life and his work caused much controversy. His most famous collection is *Leaves of Grass.*

___ 13. This Russian author was best known for his books *War and Peace* and *Anna Karenina.*

a. Charles Dickens

b. Noah Webster

c. Hans Christian Andersen

d. Pearl Buck

e. John Steinbeck

f. Samuel Clemens (Mark Twain)

g. William Shakespeare

h. Louisa May Alcott

i. Aesop

j. Ernest Hemingway

k. Leo Tolstoy

l. Walt Whitman

m. Jules Verne

Who Wrote What? ANSWER SHEET

___ 1. This man wrote books of life on the Mississippi River. Huck Finn and Tom Sawyer were two of his favorite characters.

___ 2. This French author was one of the first to write science fiction. His most famous works include *Around the World in 80 Days* and *Twenty Thousand Leagues Under the Sea.*

___ 3. This man lived in ancient Greece and was credited for writing a series of fables that all had a moral lesson.

___ 4. This Englishman was famous for many books, some of which were made into movies that did equally well. His books include *David Copperfield*, *A Christmas Carol*, and *The Adventures of Oliver Twist.*

___ 5. This American writer was best known for her book *Little Women*, a novel based on her life growing up with three sisters.

___ 6. This American writer and educator's name is often thought of as synonymous with the dictionary.

___ 7. This author received a Pulitzer Prize in 1953 for *The Old Man and the Sea.* Though he had a troubled personal life, he received great acclaim for other books, including *The Sun Also Rises, A Farewell to Arms,* and *For Whom the Bell Tolls.*

___ 8. One of the best-known American authors of the 20th century, this man from Salinas, CA, wrote many books about that area, including *Cannery Row.* Other books include *The Grapes of Wrath* and *Of Mice and Men.*

___ 9. This Danish author was best known for writing fairy tales, including *The Ugly Duckling, The Emperor's New Clothes,* and *The Little Mermaid.*

___ 10. This English author, nicknamed "The Bard of Avon," wrote dozens of plays, sonnets, and poems. Some of his most famous include *Macbeth, Hamlet,* and *Romeo and Juliet.*

___ 11. This 20th-century American author spent much of her life in China. Her most famous book is *The Good Earth.*

___ 12. This 19th-century poet was thought by many to be America's best poet, though his life and his work caused much controversy. His most famous collection is *Leaves of Grass.*

___ 13. This Russian author was best known for his books *War and Peace* and *Anna Karenina.*

f. **Samuel Clemens (Mark Twain)**

m. **Jules Verne**

i. **Aesop**

a. **Charles Dickens**

h. **Louisa May Alcott**

b. **Noah Webster**

j. **Ernest Hemingway**

e. **John Steinbeck**

c. **Hans Christian Andersen**

g. **William Shakespeare**

d. **Pearl Buck**

l. **Walt Whitman**

k. **Leo Tolstoy**

FACILITATOR: *For some participants who have read much during their lifetimes, these names will be very familiar. For others, they may be unknown. Discuss each author and their works, possibly reading short passages or showing a movie clip of those that have been made into movies or plays. Do they have a favorite author? Do they enjoy reading? Have they done any writing themselves? Would they like to write a book, a poem, or a play? What would it be about?*

The World of Music

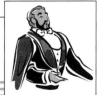

Composing, writing, and performing songs are truly art forms that we can all enjoy. We say, hum, or sing the words, making lasting memories. Most of us have not only favorite songs, but also favorite artists and we often search out music performed by them. Are any of the following musicians among your favorites?

1. This English quartet from Liverpool got its American start on the *Ed Sullivan Show*.

2. This cowboy couple's most famous song was "Happy Trails to You."

3. "God Bless America" was one of her most famous songs.

4. This songwriting duo was most famous for broadway musicals, such as *Oklahoma*, *South Pacific*, *Carousel*, and *The King and I*.

5. This man began to study the violin at the age of 6, and his "ineptness" at it later become his trademark. In reality, he was a very accomplished violinist.

6. This cultural icon is known as "The King of Rock and Roll."

7. "White Christmas" was his most famous hit.

8. This Swedish-born opera soprano singer was known as "the Swedish Nightingale."

9. Dixieland Jazz, the trumpet, and "Hello Dolly" were his trademarks.

10. This American jazz musician was known as "the King of Swing." He and his band began the Swing Era.

11. Performing in *The Jazz Singer*, this musician thrilled his audiences with his vaudvillian style and comedy from 1911 to his death in 1950.

12. Known mainly for his military marches, this composer and conductor was known as "the March King."

13. This country singer/songwriter was known for his deep voice and his black clothes. He was known as "the Man in Black."

14. This Italian singer, comedian, and actor had hits such as "That's Amore" and "Everybody Loves Somebody."

15. This is one of the best known boys' choirs in the world. They come from a well-known musical haven in Austria.

16. With his brother George, he wrote "Porgy and Bess," "I Got Rhythm," and many other Broadway hits.

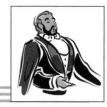

1. This English quartet from Liverpool got its American start on the *Ed Sullivan Show*.
   The Beatles

2. This cowboy couple's most famous song was "Happy Trails to You."
   Roy Rogers & Dale Evans

3. "God Bless America" was one of her most famous songs.
   Kate Smith

4. This songwriting duo was most famous for broadway musicals, such as *Oklahoma*, *South Pacific*, *Carousel,* and *The King and I.*
   Rodgers and Hammerstein

5. This man began to study the violin at the age of 6, and his "ineptness" at it later become his trademark. In reality, he was a very accomplished violinist.
   Jack Benny

6. This cultural icon is known as "The King of Rock and Roll."
   Elvis Presley

7. "White Christmas" was his most famous hit.
   Bing Crosby

8. This Swedish-born opera soprano singer was known as "the Swedish Nightingale."
   Jenny Lind

9. Dixieland Jazz, the trumpet, and "Hello Dolly" were his trademarks.
   Louis Armstrong

10. This American jazz musician was known as "the King of Swing." He and his band began the Swing Era.
    Benny Goodman

11. Performing in *The Jazz Singer*, this musician thrilled his audiences with his vaudvillian style and comedy from 1911 to his death in 1950.
    Al Jolson

12. Known mainly for his military marches, this composer and conductor was known as "the March King."
    John Philip Sousa

13. This country singer/songwriter was known for his deep voice and his black clothes. He was known as "the Man in Black."
    Johnny Cash

14. This Italian singer, comedian, and actor had hits such as "That's Amore" and "Everybody Loves Somebody."
    Dean Martin

15. This is one of the best known boys' choirs in the world. They come from a well-known musical haven in Austria.
    Vienna Boys' Choir

16. With his brother George, he wrote "Porgy and Bess," "I Got Rhythm," and many other Broadway hits.
    Ira Gershwin

FACILITATOR: *As with any music activity, this one is sure to prompt some to break out in song. Take advantage of this and plan a sing-along after completing this activity by using some of the songs of these artists. Ask participants for details on these people—when they lived, which songs they sang best, something about their lives, and so forth. Which were participants' favorite artists? What do they think it would be like to sing before thousands of people?*

Places

The word *place* is defined as "a spot or position that is or can be occupied by a person or thing." There are places of interest all around us. Tiny towns, bustling urban areas, historical sites, countries across the oceans and seas, and quiet natural areas all have qualities that make them unique and worthy of study. Perhaps you have traveled extensively in your life, or maybe you are just beginning to explore places that interest you. This section will challenge your mind as you take a "journey" through cities, states, and countries. To make your journey more interesting, keep a map or atlas handy for reference. And above all, have fun!

At the Baseball Park and on the Golf Course

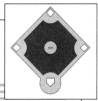

The origins of both baseball and golf date back hundreds of years. They are popular in many parts of the world and certainly rank among the favorite sports for many people in the United States. Test your knowledge of these two sports with the following activity.

1. This game is played in the middle of the baseball season with the best players from the National League playing against the best of the American League.

2. The first recorded game of golf was played in 1456 in this country.

3. Name the number of:
   a. innings in a baseball game
   b. holes in a typical golf course
   c. feet between the first and second base
   d. defensive players on a baseball field

4. The name for a score on a hole in golf where the golfer goes:
   a. one over par
   b. one under par
   c. two under par

5. How many positions on a baseball team can you name?

6. This song is traditionally played during the 7th inning of a baseball game.

7. This young player is, as of 2008, thought of by most as the best player in golf.

8. This is the seven-game contest between baseball's National League best and American League best and is played at the end of the season to determine the best team in baseball.

9. This is the number of strokes above par that a golfer will usually score on any given day.

10. This controversial baseball player broke Hank Aaron's home run record of 755 in 2007.

11. The person who typically attends to a golfer while on the course and hands him or her golf clubs.

12. This popular recording by Abbott and Costello is a classic baseball skit.

13. The oldest and perhaps the most famous golf course in the world is in Fife, Scotland, and is named this.

14. The Baseball Hall of Fame is located in this city in New York.

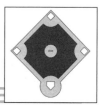

1. This game is played in the middle of the baseball season with the best players from the National League playing against the best of the American League.
    All-Star Game

2. The first recorded game of golf was played in 1456 in this country.
    Scotland

3. Name the number of:
    a. **innings in a baseball game**   9
    b. **holes in a typical golf course**   18
    c. **feet between the first and second base** 90
    d. **defensive players on a baseball field**   9

4. The name for a score on a hole in golf where the golfer goes:
    a. **one over par**   bogey
    b. **one under par**   birdie
    c. **two under par**   eagle

5. How many positions on a baseball team can you name?
    pitcher; catcher; first, second, and third baseman; shortstop; left, center, and right fielder

6. This song is traditionally played during the 7th inning of a baseball game.
    "Take Me Out to the Ball Game"

7. This young player is, as of 2008, thought of by most as the best player in golf.
    Tiger Woods

8. This is the seven-game contest between baseball's National League best and American League best and is played at the end of the season to determine the best team in baseball.
    World Series

9. This is the number of strokes above par that a golfer will usually score on any given day.
    handicap

10. This controversial baseball player broke Hank Aaron's home run record of 755 in 2007.
    Barry Bonds

11. The person who typically attends to a golfer while on the course and hands him or her golf clubs.
    caddie

12. This popular comedy routine by Abbott and Costello is a classic baseball skit.
    "Who's on First?"

13. The oldest and perhaps the most famous golf course in the world is in Fife, Scotland, and is named this.
    St. Andrews

14. The Baseball Hall of Fame is located in this city in New York.
    Cooperstown

FACILITATOR: *Many of your participants have probably played one or both of these sports. They may like to bring in pictures, bats, gloves, golf clubs, trophies, and so forth to accompany this activity. How many have played each? How many enjoy watching these sports? Who do they think the best baseball player and best golfer of all time are? How would it be to be a professional athlete? What do they think about the huge salaries paid to professional athletes? Are the athletes worth it? Are they good role models for youth today?*

At the Movies

For decades movies have been a favorite pastime for people of all ages. From early black-and-white films to the high-tech productions of today, movies are a welcome diversion from everyday life. This worksheet is about all facets of movie production.

1.   An early show, often for a bargain price.

2.   In the 1980s, this pair of movie critics became known for their movie review television show and often disagreed or argued about their views and opinions of movies.

3.   This type of theater reached its height of popularity in the 1950s and was known for its open-air style and large screens.

4.   There are many movie production companies. Can you name three?

5.   This era of motion pictures during the 1930s and '40s was known for the emergence of many of Hollywood's most glamorous and powerful stars.

6.   This awards program, which started in 1928, honors excellence in the movie industry.

7.   The creation of this device in the 1980s enabled people to watch movies in the privacy and comfort of their own homes.

8.   Which movie is widely considered the greatest film of all time? (Hint: it was produced in 1941.)

9.   Instead of the movie theater, early venues to watch movies were called what?

10. These movie clips are shown before the actual feature film begins to give the audience previews of movies to come.

11. A person who sees many movies and knows details of many films is called a what?

12. This type of film is produced by an independent filmmaker and is out of the mainstream.

13. About how much did it cost to see a movie in the 1920s? How about the 1960s? The 1980s?

14. Watching two movies in a theater back to back for the price of one is called what?

15. If a movie makes a lot of money at the box office, it is called a big hit or a what?

16. A film based on reality or historical records is called a what?

17. One of the most popular movies of all time, this 1939 film earned nearly $200 million. Adjusted for inflation, that would equal over $1 billion today.

1. An early show, often for a bargain price.
   matinee
2. In the 1980s, this pair of movie critics became known for their movie review television show and often disagreed or argued about their views and opinions of movies.
   Siskel and Ebert
3. This type of theater reached its height of popularity in the 1950s and was known for its open-air style and large screens.
   drive-in
4. There are many movie production companies. Can you name three?
   Columbia, Disney, Fox, Paramount, Sony, Universal, MGM
5. This era of motion pictures during the 1930s and '40s was known for the emergence of many of Hollywood's most glamorous and powerful stars.
   Golden Age of Hollywood
6. This awards program, which started in 1928, honors excellence in the movie industry.
   Academy Awards
7. The creation of this device in the 1980s enabled people to watch movies in the privacy and comfort of their own homes.
   VCR
8. Which movie is widely considered the greatest film of all time? (Hint: it was produced in 1941.)
   Citizen Kane
9. Instead of the movie theater, early venues to watch movies were called what?
   picture houses
10. These movie clips are shown before the actual feature film begins to give the audience previews of movies to come.
    trailers
11. A person who sees many movies and knows details of many films is called a what?
    movie buff
12. This type of film is produced by an independent filmmaker and is out of the mainstream.
    underground
13. About how much did it cost to see a movie in the 1920s? How about the 1960s? The 1980s?
    1920s: 27¢
    1960s: 90¢
    1980s: $4
14. Watching two movies in a theater back to back for the price of one is called what?
    double feature
15. If a movie makes a lot of money at the box office, it is called a big hit or a what?
    blockbuster
16. A film based on reality or historical records is called a what?
    documentary
17. One of the most popular movies of all time, this 1939 film earned nearly $200 million. Adjusted for inflation, that would equal over $1 billion today.
    Gone with the Wind

FACILITATOR: *Bring in some samples of movie boxes or movie paraphernalia to show the group. Use this worksheet to bring up discussion on the following topics: How do movies of today differ from those of yesteryear? Who is or was your favorite actor or actress? Did you enjoy silent movies; if so, which was your favorite? Have you ever met a famous actor or actress or been to a movie set?*

The A–Z of U.S. Cities

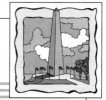

How many cities can you name around the United States for each letter of the alphabet. Examples are given on the answer sheet on the back.

A

B

C

D

E

F

G

H

I

J

K

L

M

N

O

P

Q

R

S

T

U

V

W

X

Y

Z

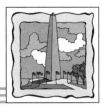

A   Akron / Aspen / Anchorage

B   Boise / Baton Rouge / Boston

C   Chicago / Cleveland / Cheyenne

D   Denver / Dallas / Detroit

E   Eugene / Evanston / El Paso

F   Fort Benning / Fort Worth / Fargo

G   Greensboro / Green Bay / Grand Rapids

H   Houston / Honolulu / Hartford

I   Indianapolis / Ithaca / Idaho Falls

J   Jefferson City / Jacksonville / Juneau

K   Kansas City / Kennebunkport / Kalamazoo

L   Las Vegas / Lexington / Little Rock

M   Milwaukee / Miami / Memphis

N   New Orleans / Nashville / Norfolk

O   Oklahoma City / Orlando / Omaha

P   Portland / Palm Springs / Phoenix

Q   Quincy / Queensboro / Quinhagak (Alaska)

R   Reno / Richmond / Rochester

S   Sacramento / Salem / Salt Lake City

T   Topeka / Tampa / Tucson

U   Union / Utica / Ukiah

V   Vail / Vancouver / Virginia Beach

W   Washington, DC / Wichita / Williamsburg

X   Xenia (Ohio) / We could not find anymore. Can you?

Y   Yukon / York / Yakima

Z   Zanesville / Zumbrota / Zion

FACILITATOR: *Be sure and use a map for this activity. Participants are sure to have a wide range of answers. Use the ones above as examples after they have named those that they can. Use the A–Z list for other topics as well.*

Early Homes of U.S. Presidents

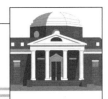

Some of the presidents of the United States got their start in poor, country houses. Others were born to wealth in places such as New York City. Some began their careers as politicians, but most worked in a variety of other jobs in places throughout the nation before turning to politics. Match the birthplaces and other locations associated with their upbringing on the left with the president on the right.

___ 1. This president spent time before the outbreak of the Revolutionary War at his Mt. Vernon home in Virginia, the state in which he was born.

___ 2. This president was born in Kentucky and moved to Indiana after his mother died when he was 10 years old.

___ 3. This president was born in Plains, Georgia, and was raised on a peanut farm.

___ 4. This president was associated with Hollywood for many years and appeared in three films over his movie star career.

___ 5. This president was born in Hyde Park, New York.

___ 6. This man was the only president born in California.

___ 7. This president was born in Lamar, Missouri, and grew up in nearby Independence as a farmer.

___ 8. This young president was born in Massachusetts and spent much of his time in his family's home in Hyannis Port.

___ 9. This president was born in Texas but grew up in Abilene, Kansas.

___ 10. This president was born in Hope, Arkansas.

___ 11. This president was born in Stonewall, Texas, in a small farmhouse.

___ 12. This president was born in New York City and lived there much of his life until his mother and first wife died on the same day, at which time he moved to the Dakota Territory.

___ 13. This president was born in New York but moved to Odessa, Texas, when he was 2 years old.

___ 14. This president was born in Nebraska, immediately moved with his mother to Illinois, and soon moved again to Grand Rapids, Michigan, where he became a football star in both high school and college.

___ 15. This president was born into a Quaker family in West Branch, Iowa, and was the son of a blacksmith.

a. Ronald Reagan

b. Richard Nixon

c. John F. Kennedy (JFK)

d. Lyndon B. Johnson (LBJ)

e. Jimmy Carter

f. George W. Bush

g. Gerald Ford

h. Abraham Lincoln

i. Harry S. Truman

j. Theodore ("Teddy") Roosevelt

k. Dwight D. Eisenhower

l. Herbert Hoover

m. George Washington

n. Bill Clinton

o. Franklin D. Roosevelt (FDR)

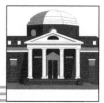

Early Homes of U.S. Presidents ANSWER SHEET

1. This president spent time before the outbreak of the Revolutionary War at his Mt. Vernon home in Virginia, the state in which he was born.

2. This president was born in Kentucky and moved to Indiana after his mother died when he was 10 years old.

3. This president was born in Plains, Georgia, and was raised on a peanut farm.

4. This president was associated with Hollywood for many years and appeared in three films over his movie star career.

5. This president was born in Hyde Park, New York.

6. This man was the only president born in California.

7. This president was born in Lamar, Missouri, and grew up in nearby Independence as a farmer.

8. This young president was born in Massachusetts and spent much of his time in his family's home in Hyannis Port.

9. This president was born in Texas but grew up in Abilene, Kansas.

10. This president was born in Hope, Arkansas.

11. This president was born in Stonewall, Texas, in a small farmhouse.

12. This president was born in New York City and lived there much of his life until his mother and first wife died on the same day, at which time he moved to the Dakota Territory.

13. This president was born in New York but moved to Odessa, Texas, when he was 2 years old.

14. This president was born in Nebraska, immediately moved with his mother to Illinois, and soon moved again to Grand Rapids, Michigan, where he became a football star in both high school and college.

15. This president was born into a Quaker family in West Branch, Iowa, and was the son of a blacksmith.

m. **George Washington**

h. **Abraham Lincoln**

e. **Jimmy Carter**

a. **Ronald Reagan**

o. **Franklin D. Roosevelt (FDR)**

b. **Richard Nixon**

i. **Harry S. Truman**

c. **John F. Kennedy (JFK)**

k. **Dwight D. Eisenhower**

n. **Bill Clinton**

d. **Lyndon B. Johnson (LBJ)**

j. **Theodore ("Teddy") Roosevelt**

f. **George W. Bush**

g. **Gerald Ford**

l. **Herbert Hoover**

FACILITATOR: *Using a map for this exercise would be helpful. How many participants have visited these places? Have they visited any of the presidential libraries? An interesting fact to point out is that approximately one-third of U.S. presidents were born in just two states—seven in Ohio (Grant, Garfield, Hayes, Harrison, McKinley, Taft, and Harding), and eight in Virginia (Washington, Jefferson, Madison, Monroe, Harrison, Tyler, Taylor, and Wilson). Why do they think this might be true?*

Strengthen Your Mind, Volume Two by Einberger & Sellick. Copyright © 2008 by Health Professions Press, Inc.

The East Coast

The East Coast is sometimes thought of as those states in the northeast. Other times, the Mid-Atlantic states are included. Even less frequently, those states from Virginia to Florida are included. All of these states, however, are geographically located on the East Coast. The following facts are all related to the East Coast states located along the Atlantic Ocean.

1. This famous ship carried pilgrims from Plymouth, England, to Plymouth, Massachusetts, in 1620.

2. This large statue in the New York Harbor serves as a welcome to all who enter.

3. Four East Coast states border Canada. Can you name any of them?

4. This huge granite stone near Atlanta is home to a flat sculpture into which is carved the figures of Robert E. Lee, Stonewall Jackson, and Jefferson Davis.

5. This city, the most populated in the United States, is often called the Big Apple.

6. This city, our nation's capital, is not actually located within any U.S. state.

7. This well-known tourist attraction borders New York and Ontario, Canada, and is made up of Horseshoe Falls and American Falls.

8. The southern part of the East Coast is particularly known for these very high winds.

9. This over 2,000-mile-long trail goes from Georgia to Maine and is hiked by thousands every year.

10. This city is the birthplace of American democracy and was the nation's first capital from 1791 to 1800.

11. All human space flight missions take off from this NASA center in Florida.

12. In 1607, this city in Virginia became the first permanent English settlement in the United States.

13. In 1492, Columbus used these three ships to sail to the East Coast.

14. Tourists from near and far visit the New England states in the Fall to see this.

15. From 1892 until 1954, this island in New York Harbor served as the immigration center for people entering the United States.

16. This large city in southeastern Florida is known as the "cruise capital of the world." It also serves as one of the most prominent U.S. links to Latin America.

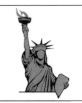

The East Coast ANSWER SHEET

1. This famous ship carried pilgrims from Plymouth, England, to Plymouth, Massachusetts, in 1620.
   Mayflower

2. This large statue in the New York Harbor serves as a welcome to all who enter.
   Statue of Liberty

3. Four East Coast states border Canada. Can you name any of them?
   Maine, New Hampshire, New York, Vermont

4. This huge granite stone near Atlanta is home to a flat sculpture into which is carved the figures of Robert E. Lee, Stonewall Jackson, and Jefferson Davis.
   Stone Mountain

5. This city, the most populated in the United States, is often called the Big Apple.
   New York City

6. This city, our nation's capital, is not actually located within any U.S. state.
   Washington, DC

7. This well-known tourist attraction borders New York and Ontario, Canada, and is made up of Horseshoe Falls and American Falls.
   Niagara Falls

8. The southern part of the East Coast is particularly known for these very high winds.
   hurricanes

9. This over 2,000-mile-long trail goes from Georgia to Maine and is hiked by thousands every year.
   Appalachian Trail

10. This city is the birthplace of American democracy and was the nation's first capital from 1791 to 1800.
    Philadelphia

11. All human space flight missions take off from this NASA center in Florida.
    Kennedy Space Center

12. In 1607, this city in Virginia became the first permanent English settlement in the United States.
    Jamestown

13. In 1492, Columbus used these three ships to sail to the East Coast.
    Niña, Pinta, Santa Maria

14. Tourists from near and far visit the New England states in the Fall to see this.
    Fall foliage

15. From 1892 until 1954, this island in New York Harbor served as the immigration center for people entering the United States.
    Ellis Island

16. This large city in southeastern Florida is known as the "cruise capital of the world." It also serves as one of the most prominent U.S. links to Latin America.
    Miami

FACILITATOR: *It can be useful to have participants point out these different locations on a map. How many of these places have they seen? Which would they like to see? Which other East Coast states or sites would they like to visit? How many of the participants were born in these states? What else is the East Coast known for? Food? Famous people? Cities? Tourist attractions?*

The High Seas

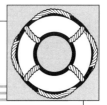

The five oceans (Arctic, Atlantic, Indian, Pacific, and Southern) cover more than two-thirds of the Earth's surface. Lesser bodies of water, such as the seas, cover part of the remaining third. These waters are used for a multitude of purposes, from serving as the water "highway" for thousands of vessels each day to serving as the setting for many wonderful books. How many of the following facts about the Earth's water can you identify?

1. This person was a castaway who spent 28 years on a remote tropical island and is the lead character in a book written by Daniel Defoe.

2. Herman Melville wrote this book about a great white whale.

3. This legendary boat was the setting for a weekly television show of the 1970s and '80s. Captain Merrill Stubing led the cast in humorous and romantic adventures.

4. This boat, which carried passengers from the 1930s to the '60s in the North Atlantic, is now a museum in Long Beach, California.

5. This was a boat commandeered by John F. Kennedy during World War II. A movie with the same name was later made of his heroic actions on this boat.

6. This very popular adventure book by Robert Louis Stevenson focused on pirates, buried gold, and buccaneers.

7. Which type of bird is most seen on the shoulders of pirates and buccaneers?

8. Though there are actually many more, we often hear about the seven seas. Can you name them?

9. What kind of boat is responsible for towing barges?

10. What would you find on a pirate flag, commonly known as the Jolly Roger?

11. The villain in the novel titled *Peter Pan* is a captain who goes by this name.

12. This British passenger ship sank tragically when it hit an iceberg in 1912.

13. This warship serves as an airbase at sea.

14. This is a small boat carried aboard a large boat and is often used for carrying passengers to shore when a boat is too large to enter a marina or harbor.

15. In 1915 during World War I, this British luxury liner was torpedoed by a German submarine, killing over 1,000 people aboard.

16. This British branch of the armed services was for over a hundred years the largest and most powerful in the world.

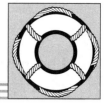

1. This person was a castaway who spent 28 years on a remote tropical island and is the lead character in a book written by Daniel Defoe.
   Robinson Crusoe

2. Herman Melville wrote this book about a great white whale.
   Moby Dick

3. This legendary boat was the setting for a weekly television show of the 1970s and '80s. Captain Merrill Stubing led the cast in humorous and romantic adventures.
   The Love Boat

4. This boat, which carried passengers from the 1930s to the '60s in the North Atlantic, is now a museum in Long Beach, California.
   Queen Mary

5. This was a boat commandeered by John F. Kennedy during World War II. A movie with the same name was later made of his heroic actions on this boat.
   PT-109

6. This very popular adventure book by Robert Louis Stevenson focused on pirates, buried gold, and buccaneers.
   Treasure Island

7. Which type of bird is most seen on the shoulders of pirates and buccaneers?
   parrot

8. Though there are actually many more, we often hear about the seven seas. Can you name them?
   Adriatic, Aegean, Arabian, Caspian, Indian, Mediterranean, Persian Gulf, Red

9. What kind of boat is responsible for towing barges?
   tugboat

10. What would you find on a pirate flag, commonly known as the Jolly Roger?
    skull and crossbones

11. The villain in the novel titled *Peter Pan* is a captain who goes by this name.
    Captain Hook

12. This British passenger ship sank tragically when it hit an iceberg in 1912.
    Titanic

13. This warship serves as an airbase at sea.
    aircraft carrier

14. This is a small boat carried aboard a large boat and is often used for carrying passengers to shore when a boat is too large to enter a marina or harbor.
    dinghy

15. In 1915 during World War I, this British luxury liner was torpedoed by a German submarine, killing over 1,000 people aboard.
    Lusitania

16. This British branch of the armed services was for over a hundred years the largest and most powerful in the world.
    Royal Navy

FACILITATOR: *The oceans and seas of the world can be the basis for many questions. A map would be helpful for this activity. Ask how many participants have been on a boat. Which type? Has anyone been on a cruise? Where to? Has anyone read any of the books listed above? If participants were stranded on a deserted island, which three things would they want with them? Whom would they like to be with on the island? Has anyone ever watched* The Love Boat *or* Gilligan's Island? *How about the movie* Peter Pan *with Robin Williams?*

Home Sweet Home

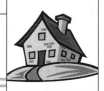

For many of us, there's no place like home! It is where we want to be, more than any other place on Earth. The following are descriptions of phrases and titles that contain the word *home*. Can you name each?

1. "Oh give me a home" is the beginning of this classic western song, now the state song of Kansas.

2. Someone who would prefer to stay at home is called a what?

3. In baseball, a batter stands at this when he's batting.

4. The science of homemaking and also a course that girls especially used to take in high school.

5. This is a relatively new agency within the federal government that was created after terrorists struck the World Trade Center.

6. Beer that is made at home is called this.

7. Rather than give away gifts that are purchased, many people would prefer to give away something that is what?

8. A person, usually a woman, who manages a household.

9. Teachers often assign this to students to be done outside of school.

10. When a country is at war, we often refer to civilians as being on the what?

11. Land claimed by settlers or squatters, such as in the Oklahoma land rush, is called a what?

12. In the "Star Spangled Banner," the United States is referred to as the "land of the free" and what?

13. The city where a person was born.

14. When a person misses being home, they are referred to as this.

15. The wage earner in a household is said to be the one who does this.

16. When a batter hits the ball over the center-field fence, he's hit a what?

17. When we fix up our houses to look better, we are making these.

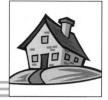

1. "Oh give me a home" is the beginning of this classic western song, now the state song of Kansas.
   "Home on the Range"

2. Someone who would prefer to stay at home is called a what?
   homebody

3. In baseball, a batter stands at this when he's batting.
   home plate

4. The science of homemaking and also a course that girls especially used to take in high school.
   home economics

5. This is a relatively new agency within the federal government that was created after terrorists struck the World Trade Center.
   Homeland Security

6. Beer that is made at home is called this.
   home brew

7. Rather than give away gifts that are purchased, many people would prefer to give away something that is what?
   homemade

8. A person, usually a woman, who manages a household.
   homemaker

9. Teachers often assign this to students to be done outside of school.
   homework

10. When a country is at war, we often refer to civilians as being on the what?
    home front

11. Land claimed by settlers or squatters, such as in the Oklahoma land rush, is called a what?
    homestead

12. In the "Star Spangled Banner," the United States is referred to as the "land of the free" and what?
    "the home of the brave"

13. The city where a person was born.
    hometown

14. When a person misses being home, they are referred to as this.
    homesick

15. The wage earner in a household is said to be the one who does this.
    brings home the bacon

16. When a batter hits the ball over the center-field fence, he's hit a what?
    home run

17. When we fix up our houses to look better, we are making these.
    home improvements

FACILITATOR: *You might want to use this activity as a time to urge participants to talk about their homes over the years—first home, favorite home, cost of homes then and now, and so forth. Also, ask which other expressions include the word* home, *such as "wait until the cows come home," "homespun," "homebound," and more. How important is home to participants? Do they like to travel, or are they homebodies? Can anyone draw a floor plan of his or her first home?*

In the Neighborhood

Neighborhoods vary from urban to farm, and suburban to rural; however each type of neighborhood has a life of its own. Regardless of the type(s) of neighborhood you grew up in, most have a variety of fun, games, and social opportunities. Read the following descriptions of neighborhood life. Can you name each item?

1. These large round hoops were popular with kids, who would swing them around their hips for fun.

2. This bill given to veterans by the military helped fund the boom in suburban housing in the 1950s.

3. Kids made these ride-on toys or "bugs" out of old apple boxes attached to roller skate wheels.

4. Kids could often be found outside playing this game, which consisted of one person designated as "it," other kids hiding, and a can.

5. These types of parties generally involve the whole neighborhood and can be held for holidays or other celebrations.

6. This type of socializing involved teenagers driving around town, often on a particular street to see friends.

7. Similar to an ice cream parlor, this type of establishment served colas, malts, and milkshakes.

8. Many children in the neighborhood joined clubs for social and educational opportunities. Try to list at least three.

9. After dinner most families would gather around this electronic device, which most households had by the end of the 1950s.

10. This person was a staple in the neighborhood and delivered milk and other dairy products to the doorstep of homes.

11. These parties made it possible to purchase popular plastic storage containers and provided an opportunity for women to socialize and meet new friends.

12. This truck had an attention-grabbing musical jingle and generally drove around after dinner.

13. This common children's game is usually played on the sidewalk and involves drawing a series of squares on which players have to jump.

14. With this type of dinner party you travel from house to house, meeting neighbors while enjoying a different dinner course at each location.

15. This television show was popular with kids in the 1970s and '80s and featured a musical host who began each show with the jingle "Won't you be my neighbor?"

16. In this form of fundraising, a person (usually a woman) makes a lunch that is "auctioned" to the highest bidder, who traditionally then has a date with or shares lunch with the woman who made it.

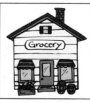

1. This large plastic ring was popular with kids, who would swing it around their hips for fun.
   hula hoop
2. This bill given to veterans by the military helped fund the boom in suburban housing in the 1950s.
   GI Bill
3. Kids made this ride-on toy or "bug" out of an old apple box attached to roller skate wheels.
   soapbox car
4. Kids could often be found outside playing this game, which consisted of one person designated as "it," other kids hiding, and a can.
   kick the can
5. These types of parties generally involve the whole neighborhood and can be held for holidays or other celebrations.
   block party
6. This type of socializing involved teenagers driving around town, often on a particular street to see friends.
   cruising
7. Similar to an ice cream parlor, this type of establishment served colas, malts, and milkshakes.
   soda shop
8. Many children in the neighborhood joined clubs for social and educational opportunities. Try to list at least three.
   Boy Scouts, Girl Scouts, 4-H, Campfire Girls
9. After dinner most families would gather around this electronic device, which most households had by the end of the 1950s.
   television
10. This person was a staple in the neighborhood and delivered milk and other dairy products to the doorstep of homes.
    milkman
11. This type of party made it possible to purchase popular plastic storage containers and provided an opportunity for women to socialize and meet new friends.
    Tupperware party
12. This truck had an attention-grabbing musical jingle and generally drove around after dinner.
    ice cream truck
13. This common children's game is usually played on the sidewalk and involves drawing a series of squares on which players have to jump.
    hopscotch
14. With this type of dinner party you travel from house to house, meeting neighbors while enjoying a different dinner course at each location.
    progressive dinner party
15. This television show was popular with kids in the 1970s and '80s and featured a musical host who began each show with the jingle "Won't you be my neighbor?"
    Mr. Rogers' Neighborhood
16. In this form of fundraising, a person (usually a woman) makes a lunch that is "auctioned" to the highest bidder, who traditionally then has a date with or shares lunch with the woman who made it.
    box social

FACILITATOR: *What type of neighborhood did you grow up in? What was daily life like? What were some transportation options in your neighborhood? Did you spend most of your time indoors or outdoors and why? Were you friends with your neighbors, or did most people stick to themselves? What kind of indoor and outdoor games did you play?*

In the Universe

Space and space travel have long fascinated people. A hundred years ago it would have been unthinkable that we could actually walk on the moon. While we know much more about the universe than we ever have, there are still so many facets of space that we know little about. Nevertheless, our interest in space is shown in both Hollywood productions and through government funding. For this worksheet, give the answer for each of the following questions.

1. The Sun, Earth, Moon, and other planets are a part of the what?

2. In the United States the government agency responsible for space research and travel.

3. The date July 21, 1969 is famous for what national event?

4. It has been widely speculated that life exists or could have existed on what other planet?

5. There are eight planets in the solar system. Can you name them?

6. When the Moon passes between the Sun and Earth.

7. In the late 1950s the Soviet Union launched this series of space missions, some carrying dogs or other animals.

8. A small body of matter that enters the Earth's atmosphere and then burns up is called a what?

9. On a clear night it is possible to see a band of white light in the sky. This sight is Earth's galaxy, which is called the what?

10. On January 28, 1986 millions of Americans witnessed the explosion of this spacecraft, which killed all seven crewmembers.

11. When a spacecraft re-enters the Earth's atmosphere, the loud, thunder-like sound that can be heard from miles away is called a what?

12. The three men on the Apollo 11 mission, the first manned mission to land on the Moon.

13. This series of fictional space films that began in the 1970s is one of the most successful film trilogies of all time.

14. A region of space that draws everything into it so that nothing can escape.

15. This term is used to explain the force that keeps the planets in rotation around the Sun.

16. When Neil Armstrong set foot on the Moon, he said this famous quote.

17. A group of stars that form a pattern in the sky is called a what?

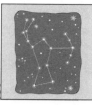

1. The Sun, Earth, Moon, and other planets are a part of the what?
   solar system
2. In the United States the government agency responsible for space research and travel.
   National Aeronautics and Space Administration
3. The date July 21, 1969 is famous for what national event?
   man first walked on the moon
4. It has been widely speculated that life exists or could have existed on what other planet?
   Mars
5. There are eight planets in the solar system. Can you name them?
   Earth, Jupiter, Mars, Mercury, Neptune, Saturn, Uranus, Venus
6. When the Moon passes between the Sun and Earth.
   solar eclipse
7. In the late 1950s the Soviet Union launched this series of space missions, some carrying dogs or other animals.
   Sputnik
8. A small body of matter that enters the Earth's atmosphere and then burns up is called a what?
   meteor or falling star
9. On a clear night it is possible to see a band of white light in the sky. This sight is Earth's galaxy, which is called the what?
   Milky Way
10. On January 28, 1986 millions of Americans witnessed the explosion of this spacecraft, which killed all seven crewmembers.
    Challenger
11. When a spacecraft re-enters the Earth's atmosphere, the loud, thunder-like sound that can be heard from miles away is called a what?
    sonic boom
12. The three men on the Apollo 11 mission, the first manned mission to land on the Moon.
    Neil Armstrong, Edwin "Buzz" Aldrin, Michael Collins
13. This series of fictional space films that began in the 1970s is one of the most successful film trilogies of all time.
    Star Wars
14. A region of space that draws everything into it so that nothing can escape.
    black hole
15. This term is used to explain the force that keeps the planets in rotation around the Sun
    gravity
16. When Neil Armstrong set foot on the Moon, he said this famous quote.
    "That's one small step for man, one giant leap for mankind."
17. A group of stars that form a pattern in the sky is called a what?
    constellation

FACILITATOR: *Depending on the interests of the group, this activity could be steered in a number of different directions. How much do participants know about the Milky Way? Names of constellations? Descriptions of the planets? Another direction would be to discuss the different things that fly—kites, birds, helicopters, and so forth. Or yet another direction would be to talk about particpants' experiences flying. When and where was their first trip on a plane? Have they ever been on a small plane? Which airline do they like best? How much do they think a ticket to certain places would cost? You might want to bring in some ads from the travel section of a magazine or newspaper to share.*

Legendary Places

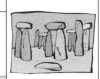

The setting for a legend is often a very important part of the story. Some settings are based on real places, some on imaginary ones. In which legendary place did the following books, movies, or television shows take place? Match the tale on the left with the location on the right.

___ 1. Frank Baum's book, *The Wizard of* . . . .

___ 2. Robin Hood's tales often take place in this forest.

___ 3. The plantation in *Gone with the Wind*.

___ 4. Plato wrote about this mysterious island in the Atlantic Ocean.

___ 5. Ponce de Leon supposedly discovered these "healing waters."

___ 6. King Arthur and his knights sat at a round table in this location.

___ 7. The tales of Dracula often take place here.

___ 8. This mystical paradise on Earth is described by James Hilton in *The Lost Horizon*.

___ 9. This is where Alice lives in Lewis Carroll's novel, *Alice in* . . . .

___ 10. Sherlock Holmes lived at this London address.

___ 11. This fictional city is the home of Batman.

___ 12. J.R.R. Tolkein's novels *The Hobbit* and *The Lord of the Rings* take place here.

___ 13. The phrase "The plane, the plane" introduced this weekly television show.

___ 14. Ichabod Crane lived here in this "legend."

___ 15. *Gunsmoke*, a long-running western television show, took place here.

___ 16. Bigfoot, also known as Sasquatch, supposedly lives in this part of the country.

___ 17. Santa's workshop is located here.

___ 18. Some say a monster lives in this lake in Scotland.

a. Transylvania

b. Gotham City

c. Wonderland

d. Sherwood Forest

e. *Fantasy Island*

f. Dodge City

g. Loch Ness

h. Lost City of Atlantis

i. Pacific Northwest

j. The Fountain of Youth

k. Sleepy Hollow

l. 221B Baker Street

m. Oz

n. Shangri-La

o. Middle Earth

p. North Pole

q. Tara

r. Camelot

Legendary Places ANSWER SHEET

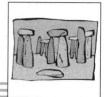

1. Frank Baum's book, *The Wizard of . . . .*   **m. Oz**

2. Robin Hood's tales often take place in this forest.   **d. Sherwood Forest**

3. The plantation in *Gone with the Wind*.   **q. Tara**

4. Plato wrote about this mysterious island in the Atlantic Ocean.   **h. Lost City of Atlantis**

5. Ponce de Leon supposedly discovered these "healing waters."   **j. The Fountain of Youth**

6. King Arthur and his knights sat at a round table in this location.   **r. Camelot**

7. The tales of Dracula often take place here.   **a. Transylvania**

8. This mystical paradise on Earth is described by James Hilton in *The Lost Horizon*. **n. Shangri-La**

9. This is where Alice lives in Lewis Carroll's novel, *Alice in . . . .*   **c. Wonderland**

10. Sherlock Holmes lived at this London address.   **l. 221B Baker Street**

11. This fictional city is the home of Batman.   **b. Gotham City**

12. J.R.R. Tolkein's novels *The Hobbit* and *The Lord of the Rings* take place here.   **o. Middle Earth**

13. The phrase "The plane, the plane" introduced this weekly television show.   **e. *Fantasy Island***

14. Ichabod Crane lived here in this "legend."   **k. Sleepy Hollow**

15. *Gunsmoke*, a long-running western television show, took place here.   **f. Dodge City**

16. Bigfoot, also known as Sasquatch, supposedly lives in this part of the country.   **i. Pacific Northwest**

17. Santa's workshop is located here.   **p. North Pole**

18. Some say a monster lives in this lake in Scotland.   **g. Loch Ness**

FACILITATOR: *These locations are based on legend. Ask participants how many exist as real places? Have they read these stories or seen these television shows or movies? What about Bigfoot? Does he really exist? Does the Loch Ness monster exist? Has anyone been to this lake in Scotland? Is there really a Camelot? How about a fountain of youth? What about Robin Hood? Is it right to take from the rich to give to the poor?*

Strengthen Your Mind, Volume Two by Einberger & Sellick. Copyright © 2008 by Health Professions Press, Inc.

Main Street, USA

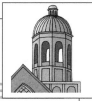

The center of many American towns is a busy place. With people, businesses, restaurants, and government buildings there is always something to do on Main Street. This sheet will take you back to life in downtown Americana, where you might just run into some of your friends or neighbors! Can you name each item described below?

1. The center of most towns is commonly marked by some type of structure. Can you name one?

2. In most county seats, the town square is located in front of this building.

3. In America, a *town square* refers to an open space in the center of town for public gathering. What is this space called in Spain? Italy? France?

4. Main street is a common location for these organized groups of people who march together to celebrate an event or holiday.

5. These tall, chiming structures keep time and often mark the center of town.

6. Many towns have similar street names, yet there is one street name that is more popular than any other. Can you name it?

7. Created in 1912, this device made it possible for multiple cars to pass through an intersection in an orderly manner.

8. Most downtown areas feature this membership organization that offers "mixers" and is intended to support and promote local business.

9. This type of celebration showcases the flair of a neighborhood and features food, crafts, and other goods for sale.

10. On many main streets parking is not free. This device is used to collect money in exchange for parking time.

11. *Street* is a common generic name given to roadways, but it is not the only name used. List three other types of roadways.

12. This famous amusement park in Los Angeles features "Main Street USA" as one of the many themed areas in the park.

13. Many downtown areas have vendors who offer street food. What is the most common food sold out of a cart?

14. This pole with red and white stripes advertises haircutting services and has been used in various forms since the 1700s.

15. Where the headquarters of a city administration is located.

16. A meeting in which the entire neighborhood or city is invited to discuss issues that relate to the community.

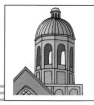

1. The center of most towns is commonly marked by some type of structure. Can you name one?
   fountain, well, statue, monument

2. In most county seats, the town square is located in front of this building.
   county courthouse

3. In America, a *town square* refers to an open space in the center of town for public gathering. What is this space called in Spain? Italy? France?
   plaza, piazza, place

4. Main street is a common location for these organized groups of people who march together to celebrate an event or holiday.
   parade

5. These tall, chiming structures keep time and often mark the center of town.
   clock tower

6. Many towns have similar street names, yet there is one street name that is more popular than any other. Can you name it?
   Second Street

7. Created in 1912, this device made it possible for multiple cars to pass through an intersection in an orderly manner.
   traffic signal

8. Most downtown areas feature this membership organization that offers "mixers" and is intended to support and promote local business.
   Chamber of Commerce

9. This type of celebration showcases the flair of a neighborhood and features food, crafts, and other goods for sale.
   street fair

10. On many main streets parking is not free. This device is used to collect money in exchange for parking time.
    parking meter

11. *Street* is a common generic name given to roadways, but it is not the only name used. List three other types of roadways.
    road, lane, circle, drive, avenue, court, boulevard

12. This famous amusement park in Los Angeles features "Main Street USA" as one of the many themed areas in the park.
    Disneyland

13. Many downtown areas have vendors who offer street food. What is the most common food sold out of a cart?
    hot dogs

14. This pole with red and white stripes advertises haircutting services and has been used in various forms since the 1700s.
    barber pole

15. Where the headquarters of a city administration is located.
    town (or city) hall

16. A meeting in which the entire neighborhood or city is invited to discuss issues that relate to the community.
    town meeting

FACILITATOR: *It is likely that this sheet will bring up discussion about participants' hometowns. Where is each person from? How many are from the city? How many are from the country? How does town life in the United States differ from town life abroad? What qualities and amenities should a good town have? If you were going to plan a city, what businesses would you be sure to include?*

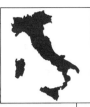

Nicknames and Historical Names of Countries around the World

People use nicknames as substitutes for names of countries around the world. Also, throughout history country names have changed as a result of war, religious influence, revolution, and so forth. The names on the left are either a nickname or historical name. Can you match the name on the left to the country on the right?

___ 1. The Jewel in the Crown   a. Ireland

___ 2. Home to the Olympics   b. China

___ 3. La République   c. Spain

___ 4. The Emerald Isle   d. Taiwan

___ 5. Mesopotamia   e. The Philippines

___ 6. Persia   f. Australia

___ 7. The Cradle of Civilization   g. Japan

___ 8. The Red Dragon   h. Iran

___ 9. Land of Chocolate and Cuckoo Clocks   i. India

___ 10. Hispania   j. Israel

___ 11. Land of the Huns   k. The Netherlands

___ 12. Pearl of the Orient   l. Italy

___ 13. Siam   m. France

___ 14. Formosa   n. Switzerland

___ 15. The Boot   o. Thailand

___ 16. Kiwiland   p. New Zealand

___ 17. Land of the Rising Sun   q. Iraq

___ 18. The Holy Land   r. Greece

___ 19. Down Under   s. Hungary

___ 20. Holland   t. Greece

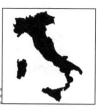

1.	The Jewel in the Crown	**i.**	**India**
2.	Home to the Olympics	**t.**	**Greece**
3.	La République	**m.**	**France**
4.	The Emerald Isle	**a.**	**Ireland**
5.	Mesopotamia	**q.**	**Iraq**
6.	Persia	**h.**	**Iran**
7.	The Cradle of Civilization	**r.**	**Greece**
8.	The Red Dragon	**b.**	**China**
9.	Land of Chocolate and Cuckoo Clocks	**n.**	**Switzerland**
10.	Hispania	**c.**	**Spain**
11.	Land of the Huns	**s.**	**Hungary**
12.	Pearl of the Orient	**e.**	**The Philippines**
13.	Siam	**o.**	**Thailand**
14.	Formosa	**d.**	**Taiwan**
15.	The Boot	**l.**	**Italy**
16.	Kiwiland	**p.**	**New Zealand**
17.	Land of the Rising Sun	**g.**	**Japan**
18.	The Holy Land	**j.**	**Israel**
19.	Down Under	**f.**	**Australia**
20.	Holland	**k.**	**The Netherlands**

FACILITATOR: *Be sure and use a map for this activity, pointing out each country (or having participants do so). What else do they know about the country? Where do they think the nickname came from? Do they know of any other country nicknames? Can they name any other country whose name was changed? Do they know why the country name was changed?*

On the Map

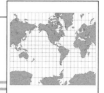

Maps have been around for hundreds of years. They were first used for property lines, tax collecting, and voyages through familiar territories. There was little interest in "the land beyond." Today, however, maps are used for a variety of purposes, from navigating waters to identifying geological features. How much do you know about maps? Can you identify the following features?

1. The study of making maps is called what?

2. This feature lets us know that 1 inch equals 100 miles on a map.

3. A collection of maps, usually in book form, is called what?

4. The imaginary line that runs halfway between the North Pole and South Pole is called the what?

5. A navigational instrument used for finding directions (N, S, E, and W) is called what?

6. A key to the color codes and symbols on a map is called a what?

7. This is the study of Earth's surface. This type of map identifies bodies of water, mountains, and so forth.

8. A three-dimensional round map is called a what?

9. How many types of maps can you name?

10. When we want to know the best way to get somewhere, we want to know the best what?

11. On the 6 o'clock news, we often see this type of map, which tells us whether or not there is rain in the forecast.

12. This company is the best-known producer of maps of all kinds.

13. Until 1991 this was the largest country on a world map.

14. This line gives the location of a place on Earth north and south of the equator.

15. This line gives the location of a place on Earth east and west of the equator.

16. This scientific division of the federal government, the U.S.G.S., studies the landscape of the United States and its natural resources. What do the initials stand for?

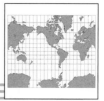

On the Map ANSWER SHEET

1. The study of making maps is called what?
   cartography

2. This feature lets us know that 1 inch equals 100 miles on a map.
   scale

3. A collection of maps, usually in book form, is called what?
   atlas

4. The imaginary line that runs halfway between the North Pole and South Pole is called the what?
   equator

5. A navigational instrument used for finding directions (N, S, E, and W) is called what?
   compass

6. A key to the color codes and symbols on a map is called a what?
   legend

7. This is the study of Earth's surface. This type of map identifies bodies of water, mountains, and so forth.
   topography

8. A three-dimensional round map is called a what?
   globe

9. How many types of maps can you name?
   topographic, climate, physical, political, road, geological

10. When we want to know the best way to get somewhere, we want to know the best what?
    route

11. On the 6 o'clock news, we often see this type of map, which tells us whether or not there is rain in the forecast.
    weather map

12. This company is the best-known producer of maps of all kinds.
    Rand McNally

13. Until 1991 this was the largest country on a world map.
    U.S.S.R. (Soviet Union)

14. This line gives the location of a place on Earth north and south of the equator.
    latitude

15. This line gives the location of a place on Earth east and west of the equator.
    longitude

16. This scientific division of the federal government, the U.S.G.S., studies the landscape of the United States and its natural resources. What do the initials stand for?
    United States Geological Survey

FACILITATOR: This is a great activity for which to bring in a variety of maps, from roadmaps to globes. Ask people to locate certain places on the map. Ask for a city west of Rome or an ocean west of San Francisco. What types of maps have participants used? How often do they use a map? Have they ever used a compass in an attempt to figure out their location? How close have they been to the equator?

On the Road

Road trips are a staple of American life. Many families have tried a road trip for vacation at some point. Between long hours on the road, arguments among the kids, and endless fast food it is no wonder that many funny stories are created "on the road."

1. This type of gasoline was phased out in the 1970s because of its potentially harmful side effects.

2. Beginning in the 1930s, this route became popular for individuals seeking prosperity in the west.

3. This road runs through much of Nevada and is known as the "Loneliest Road in America."

4. These signs were popular with motorists and advertised a brand of shaving lotion through a series of sequential signs.

5. Early gas stations featured these items that sat atop gas pumps and were lighted to advertise a brand of gasoline.

6. This annual contest to determine the fuel efficiency of various automobiles was held from 1936 to 1968.

7. In 1929, this device was invented, which allowed drivers to listen to broadcasts and music while driving.

8. Gas prices have risen steadily over the years. How much was a gallon of gas in the 1950s? The 1970s? The 1990s?

9. Driving this highway will take you all the way from Alaska to the southern tip of Argentina.

10. In the 1940s, the advent of this type of food service enabled people to order and receive their food without getting out of their car.

11. Instead of their current name, early gas stations were called what?

12. Up until the 1970s most gas stations had an attendant who would pump gas for you, check your oil, and clean your windows. Although rare today, this type of service is called what?

13. A family road trip meant many hours in the car. List some of the games that kids and parents play to pass the time.

14. List three or more current brands of gasoline or gas stations.

15. Can you list any brands of gas stations that have gone out of business?

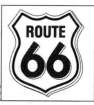

1. This type of gasoline was phased out in the 1970s because of its potentially harmful side effects.
    ethyl

2. Beginning in the 1930s, this route became popular for individuals seeking prosperity in the west.
    Route 66

3. This road runs through much of Nevada and is known as the "Loneliest Road in America."
    Route 50

4. These signs were popular with motorists and advertised a brand of shaving lotion through a series of sequential signs.
    Burma Shave

5. Early gas stations featured these items that sat atop gas pumps and were lighted to advertise a brand of gasoline.
    gas globes

6. This annual contest to determine the fuel efficiency of various automobiles was held from 1936 to 1968.
    Mobil Economy Run

7. In 1929, this device was invented, which allowed drivers to listen to broadcasts and music while driving.
    car radio

8. Gas prices have risen steadily over the years. How much was a gallon of gas in the 1950s? The 1970s? The 1990s?
    1950s: 27¢
    1970s: 36¢
    1990s: $1.16

9. Driving this highway will take you all the way from Alaska to the southern tip of Argentina.
    Pan-American Highway

10. In the 1940s, the advent of this type of food service enabled people to order and receive their food without getting out of their car.
    drive-through (or drive-thru; also called a drive-in)

11. Instead of their current name, early gas stations were called what?
    filling stations

12. Up until the 1970s most gas stations had an attendant who would pump gas for you, check your oil, and clean your windows. Although rare today, this type of service is called what?
    full-service

13. A family road trip meant many hours in the car. List some of the games that kids and parents play to pass the time.
    alphabet game; license plate game; car bingo; I spy; rock, paper, scissors

14. List three or more current brands of gasoline or gas stations.
    Texaco, Shell, ARCO, Chevron, Exxon, BP, Mobil, Valero

15. Can you list any brands of gas stations that have gone out of business?
    Gilmore, Gulf, Enco

FACILITATOR: *Bring several maps to use for discussion with the worksheet and ask the following questions for discussion: What types of road trips have you been on? To what locations? How did you pass the time in the car? Where did you stay at night? Did you take road trips as a child? How about as an adult? What is the best part about being on the road? What part do you like the least?*

Out in the Cold

Brrrrr . . . . Whether winter or summer, there are places throughout the world that see extremely cold temperatures. Yet cool weather does not seem to keep people from enjoying sports and outdoor life. After all, there is nothing like enjoying a good snowball fight or ice-skating on a frozen pond. Read each question and give an answer (and drink some hot cocoa while you read!).

1. Which continent is considered the coldest on Earth?

2. If a person stays out in the cold unprotected for too long, he or she is in danger of developing this condition on his or her extremities.

3. When it snows on Christmas Day, it is called a what?

4. This day marks the shortest day and longest night of the year as well as the beginning of the winter season.

5. A large mass of slow moving ice frequently found in the polar regions is called a what?

6. In the Southern Hemisphere, these three months are the coldest time of year.

7. Two names are used to personify winter. Can you name them both?

8. The winter Olympics are held every four years. List at least two locations where they have been held in past years.

9. Every March this famous sled dog race is run from Anchorage to Nome, Alaska.

10. These nighttime natural light displays are visible in the northern and southern polar regions.

11. On July 21, 1983, the coldest temperature ever recorded (–129 degrees Fahrenheit) occurred here.

12. In the continental United States, which major city has the lowest daily mean temperature?

13. In places where winter lasts for many months and sunlight is sparse, people may begin to feel depressed. This is otherwise known as having the what?

14. Each Groundhog Day the residents of this city in Pennsylvania gather for a community celebration to see if their famous groundhog sees its shadow, which will mean six more weeks of winter.

15. Ninety-eight percent of this cold continent is covered by ice.

16. There are many sports that are played in the cold. Can you name three?

Out in the Cold ANSWER SHEET

1. Which continent is considered the coldest on Earth?
   Antarctica

2. If a person stays out in the cold unprotected for too long, he or she is in danger of developing this condition on his or her extremities.
   frostbite

3. When it snows on Christmas Day, it is called a what?
   white Christmas

4. This day marks the shortest day and longest night of the year as well as the beginning of the winter season.
   winter solstice

5. A large mass of slow moving ice frequently found in the polar regions is called a what?
   glacier

6. In the Southern Hemisphere, these three months are the coldest time of year.
   June, July, August

7. Two names are used to personify winter. Can you name them both?
   Father Winter or Old Man Winter

8. The winter Olympics are held every four years. List at least two locations where they have been held in past years.
   Torino, Italy; Salt Lake City, Utah; Nagano, Japan; Lillehammer, Norway; Albertville, France; Calgary, Canada; Sarajevo, Yugoslavia; Lake Placid, New York; Innsbruck, Austria; and so forth

9. Every March this famous sled dog race is run from Anchorage to Nome, Alaska.
   the Iditarod

10. These nighttime natural light displays are visible in the northern and southern polar regions.
    Northern or Southern Lights

11. On July 21, 1983, the coldest temperature ever recorded (−129 degrees Fahrenheit) occurred here.
    Vostock, Antarctica

12. In the continental United States, which major city has the lowest daily mean temperature?
    Milwaukee, Wisconsin (47.5 degrees Fahrenheit)

13. In places where winter lasts for many months and sunlight is sparse, people may begin to feel depressed. This is otherwise known as having the what?
    winter blues

14. Each Groundhog Day the residents of this city in Pennsylvania gather for a community celebration to see if their famous groundhog sees its shadow, which will mean six more weeks of winter.
    Punxsutawney

15. Ninety-eight percent of this cold continent is covered by ice.
    Antarctica

16. There are many sports that are played in the cold. Can you name three?
    hockey, ice-skating, ice-climbing, bob-sledding, skiing, sled dog racing, snow-shoeing, cross-country skiing

FACILITATOR: A map will be useful for this worksheet. Find the places listed in the questions above, and try to find other places known for their cold weather on the map. Some questions to ask include: Do you prefer living in a cold or hot climate? What is the coldest temperature you have experienced? Do/did you enjoy any cold weather sports? How do you pass the time when it is too cold to go outside?

People and Places

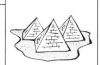

We often associate certain people with particular places—Adam and Eve with the Garden of Eden, Gandhi with India. Each of the following people listed on the left can be closely associated with a place listed on the right. Can you match them?

___ 1. St. Patrick   a. New York

___ 2. Brigham Young   b. San Simeon, California

___ 3. John Brown   c. Krypton

___ 4. William Shakespeare   d. Arkansas

___ 5. Fiorella LaGuardia   e. Dayton, Ohio

___ 6. Tom Sawyer and Huck Finn   f. Ireland

___ 7. Wright Brothers   g. Harpers Ferry ("smoldering in the grave")

___ 8. King Tutankhamun   h. Cleveland, Ohio

___ 9. Leland Stanford   i. Mississippi River

___ 10. William Randolph Hearst   j. Stratford on Avon, England

___ 11. John D. Rockefeller   k. Salt Lake City, Utah

___ 12. Andrew Carnegie   l. Piedmont, Virginia

___ 13. Superman   m. Valley of the Kings, Egypt

___ 14. Sam Walton   n. San Francisco, California

___ 15. Thomas Jefferson   o. Braddock, Pennsylvania

1. St. Patrick   f. **Ireland**

2. Brigham Young   k. **Salt Lake City, Utah**

3. John Brown   g. **Harpers Ferry ("smoldering in the grave")**

4. William Shakespeare   j. **Stratford on Avon, England**

5. Fiorella LaGuardia   a. **New York**

6. Tom Sawyer and Huck Finn   i. **Mississippi River**

7. Wright Brothers   e. **Dayton, Ohio**

8. King Tutankhamun   m. **Valley of the Kings, Egypt**

9. Leland Stanford   n. **San Francisco, California**

10. William Randolph Hearst   b. **San Simeon, California**

11. John D. Rockefeller   h. **Cleveland, Ohio**

12. Andrew Carnegie   o. **Braddock, Pennsylvania**

13. Superman   c. **Krypton**

14. Sam Walton   d. **Arkansas**

15. Thomas Jefferson   l. **Piedmont, Virginia**

FACILITATOR: *This worksheet is likely to bring up discussion about how and why these people are related to the places listed. What is the story behind each of these people? How many of these people have monuments or some other marker in recognition of their relation to a place? Use a map and find these locations. Can you find other places that are associated with people?*

Places Animals Live

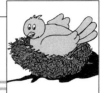

Like people, animals enjoy the comforts of home. For some it is a nest high in a tree, for others it is a network of tunnels underground. Perhaps you have even had some animals make their homes near your house, whether you welcomed them or not! For this worksheet, read each description and give the name of the animal home. If you need help, choose from the list of answers on the bottom of the page.

1. A place where birds lay their eggs and raise their young.

2. Animals that are marsupials carry their young in this.

3. Bears hibernate in this place.

4. Spiders spin these to live in and catch prey.

5. On a farm chickens live in this.

6. Bees make their home and raise their young in this.

7. A group of ants live underground in a what?

8. A name for a network of tunnels that badgers live in.

9. The name of the den where otters make their home.

10. An enclosure for dogs is called a what?

11. A small outdoor enclosure where pigs live and eat.

12. A family of snakes lives in the ground in a what?

13. A mole lives underground in a what?

14. Foxes, wolves, and tigers all make their homes in a what?

15. Beavers make their home from branches and mud and it is called a what?

16. Rabbits make their home underground in a what?

17. Bats raise their young and sleep in this.

18. A squirrel's home is made of out of twigs and leaves and is commonly called a nest or a what?

Choices: lair, sett, cave, lodge, kennel, holt, sty, nest, drey, nest, den, pouch, web, burrow, tunnel, coop, colony, hive

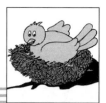

Places Animals Live ANSWER SHEET

1. A place where birds lay their eggs and raise their young.
   nest

2. Animals that are marsupials carry their young in this.
   pouch

3. Bears hibernate in this place.
   den

4. Spiders spin these to live in and catch prey.
   web

5. On a farm chickens live in this.
   coop

6. Bees make their home and raise their young in this.
   hive

7. A group of ants live underground in a what?
   colony

8. A name for a network of tunnels that badgers live in.
   sett

9. The name of the den where otters make their home.
   holt

10. An enclosure for dogs is called a what?
    kennel

11. A small outdoor enclosure where pigs live and eat.
    sty

12. A family of snakes lives in the ground in a what?
    nest

13. A mole lives underground in a what?
    tunnel

14. Foxes, wolves, and tigers all make their homes in a what?
    lair

15. Beavers make their home from branches and mud and it is called a what?
    lodge

16. Rabbits make their home underground in a what?
    burrow

17. Bats raise their young and sleep in this.
    cave

18. A squirrel's home is made of out of twigs and leaves and is commonly called a nest or a what?
    drey

FACILITATOR: *Use this worksheet for discussion on animals. From the list above, which animals would you welcome in your yard? Which would you try to get rid of? How many of these animal houses have you seen or watched animals build? Which animals live alone and which live with a family or in a group?*

Strengthen Your Mind, Volume Two by Einberger & Sellick. Copyright © 2008 by Health Professions Press, Inc.

Places Associated with the Seasons

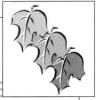

There is nothing like being inside a warm ski cabin during the winter, or enjoying a cold pool during the hot summer. There are certain places that we associate with each of the seasons. Take a quick trip around the calendar as you experience each of the seasons in this worksheet.

1. This Perry Como song produced in the 1950s croons "There's no place like _____ for the holidays."

2. Where do birds commonly migrate for Winter?

3. Where do most snowbirds tend to spend Winter?

4. This annual Spring festival in Washington, DC, commemorates the 1912 gift of Japanese Cherry Trees to the city.

5. Late Summer to Fall is known as hurricane season in these regions.

6. Many people travel during Winter to escape the cold. List three popular destinations known for warm weather during Winter in the United States.

7. During Winter, many children dream of this place, where Santa's elves are busy making toys.

8. New Year's Eve brings people out into Winter cold to celebrate. Where is the nation's largest New Year's celebration?

9. This large Arizona lake is located on the Colorado River and is one of the most popular destinations for college students on Spring break.

10. During Fall season, many families enjoy taking children to this place for hayrides and to hunt for pumpkins.

11. This region of the United States is especially known for the beautiful colors of foliage during Fall.

12. The United States is home to some premier ski resorts, a popular place to visit in Winter. List at least three.

13. Each Spring the annual Easter egg roll is held at this "home" in Washington, DC.

14. Perhaps the largest and most famous Christmas tree lighting in the United States, this one has been taking place since 1933.

15. For many Americans Summer means spending long days at the beach. List three popular beaches.

16. Every New Year's Day, millions turn on the television to watch the Rose Parade, which is held in this city.

Places Associated with the Seasons ANSWER SHEET

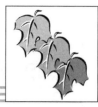

1. This Perry Como song produced in the 1950s croons "There's no place like _____ for the holidays."
   home

2. Where do birds commonly migrate for Winter?
   south

3. Where do most snowbirds tend to spend Winter?
   Florida or Arizona

4. This annual Spring festival in Washington, DC, commemorates the 1912 gift of Japanese Cherry Trees to the city.
   Cherry Blossom Festival

5. Late Summer to Fall is known as hurricane season in these regions.
   Caribbean, Mexico, southern United States

6. Many people travel during Winter to escape the cold. List three popular destinations known for warm weather during Winter in the United States.
   Hawaii, Mexico, South America, Florida

7. During Winter, many children dream of this place, where Santa's elves are busy making toys.
   North Pole

8. New Year's Eve brings people out into Winter cold to celebrate. Where is the nation's largest New Year's celebration?
   New York's Times Square

9. This large Arizona lake is located on the Colorado River and is one of the most popular destinations for college students on Spring break.
   Lake Havasu

10. During Fall season, many families enjoy taking children to this place for hayrides and to hunt for pumpkins.
    pumpkin patch

11. This region of the United States is especially known for the beautiful colors of foliage during Fall.
    New England

12. The United States is home to some premier ski resorts, a popular place to visit in Winter. List at least three.
    Vail, CO; Aspen, CO; Park City, UT; Squaw Valley, CA; Mammoth, CA; Mt. Hood, OR

13. Each Spring the annual Easter egg roll is held at this "home" in Washington, DC.
    White House

14. Perhaps the largest and most famous Christmas tree lighting in the United States, this one has been taking place since 1933.
    Rockefeller Center

15. For many Americans Summer means spending long days at the beach. List three popular beaches.
    Myrtle Beach, Cape Cod, Coronado, Venice Beach, South Beach, Malibu

16. Every New Year's Day, millions turn on the television to watch the Rose Parade, which is held in this city.
    Pasadena, California

FACILITATOR: Use this worksheet to encourage discussion about special aspects of each season. Are there special places that participants visit during Spring, Summer, Winter, or Fall? Has anyone been to any of the events listed above? Which season is their favorite? Why?

Places that Are Also Things

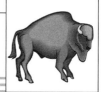

These cities, counties, and countries all have double meanings. Whether the place was named after a thing, or vice versa, enjoy identifying these well-known locations. It may be helpful to have a dictionary, map, or atlas available to check your answers.

1. This city in Georgia is also the name of a type of ecosystem with large prairies and widely spaced trees.

2. This city in New York is also the name of a large four-legged, hoofed mammal.

3. This country is also the name of a poultry bird.

4. This large city in Ohio shares its name with an explorer who is generally known for his voyages to North America.

5. This city in Arizona is also the name of an elevated area of land, usually with steep, cliff-like sides and a flat top.

6. This large, urban county located in California is also the name of one of the most popular citrus fruits to eat.

7. This city in Colorado also refers to the name of a large rock.

8. This large city in Arizona is also the name of a mythological bird that can be reborn.

9. This city in Texas is also the name of a type of plant that is native to the southern part of the United States and Mexico.

10. This city in Colorado is also the name of a home made from adobe.

11. This large South American country is also another name for a spicy addition to many foods.

12. This southwestern city in Alabama is also the name of a toy or piece of art that is hung overhead.

13. This small city in the northeastern part of Maine is also the term used for a wild reindeer.

14. This well-known city in Rhode Island is also a religious term for *love given by God*.

15. This town in Nebraska is also the name of a popular car made by Ford Motor Company.

Places that Are Also Things ANSWER SHEET

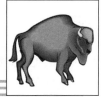

1. This city in Georgia is also the name of a type of ecosystem with large prairies and widely spaced trees.
   Savannah

2. This city in New York is also the name of a large four-legged, hoofed mammal.
   Buffalo

3. This country is also the name of a poultry bird.
   Turkey

4. This large city in Ohio shares its name with an explorer who is generally known for his voyages to North America.
   Columbus

5. This city in Arizona is also the name of an elevated area of land, usually with steep, cliff-like sides and a flat top.
   Mesa

6. This large, urban county located in California is also the name of one of the most popular citrus fruits to eat.
   Orange

7. This city in Colorado also refers to the name of a large rock.
   Boulder

8. This large city in Arizona is also the name of a mythological bird that can be reborn.
   Phoenix

9. This city in Texas is also the name of a type of plant that is native to the southern part of the United States and Mexico.
   Mesquite

10. This city in Colorado is also the name of a home made from adobe.
    Pueblo

11. This large South American country is also another name for a spicy addition to many foods.
    Chile

12. This southwestern city in Alabama is also the name of a toy or piece of art that is hung overhead.
    Mobile

13. This small city in the northeastern part of Maine is also the term used for a wild reindeer.
    Caribou

14. This well-known city in Rhode Island is also a religious term for *love given by God*.
    Providence

15. This town in Nebraska is also the name of a popular car made by Ford Motor Company.
    Lincoln

FACILITATOR: *Bring in a world map or a map of the United States and try to locate each of these places. Some questions to ask of participants: Are there any other locations that have double meanings? Why do you think these places were given these names? Do geography, wildlife, or other unique attributes of a place affect the name it's given?*

Strengthen Your Mind, Volume Two by Einberger & Sellick. Copyright © 2008 by Health Professions Press, Inc.

Settings of Famous Events

There are places all over the world that are known for a particular event that may have taken place only once or that perhaps takes place each year. Many of the places would be relatively unknown by most of us, if not for these events. How many of these sites can you name?

1. This grass track in Franklin, Kentucky, near the Tennessee border is home to many famous horse races each year.

2. A famous 500-mile auto race takes place here each Memorial Day.

3. Lincoln gave one of his most famous addresses on this battlefield in Pennsylvania during the Civil War.

4. A devastating earthquake and fire took place here in 1906.

5. In 1903, the Wright Brothers put this place in North Carolina on the map.

6. A grass court at this court in England is home to one of the four major world tennis events.

7. The running of the bulls takes place in this town in Spain each year.

8. The Grand Ole Opry in this city hosts the Country Music Association awards.

9. The famous New Year's Day Rose Bowl Parade takes place here.

10. In the 19th century, Texas fought a courageous battle at this location against the Republic of Mexico in their struggle for independence.

11. General Lee surrendered here to General Grant to end the Civil War.

12. The London Bridge was moved in 1971 from London, England, to this location in Arizona, USA.

13. President Lincoln was shot at this theater in Washington, DC.

14. American colonists destroyed many crates of tea in this harbor.

15. Mrs. O'Leary's cow kicked over a bucket to start a fire in this city.

16. The Pilgrims landed here in 1607 on the Mayflower.

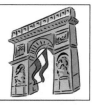

1. This grass track in Franklin, Kentucky, near the Tennessee border is home to many famous horse races each year.
   Kentucky Downs

2. A famous 500-mile auto race takes place here each Memorial Day.
   Indianapolis Motor Speedway

3. Lincoln gave one of his most famous addresses on this battlefield in Pennsylvania during the Civil War.
   Gettysburg

4. A devastating earthquake and fire took place here in 1906.
   San Francisco

5. In 1903, the Wright Brothers put this place in North Carolina on the map.
   Kitty Hawk

6. A grass court at this court in England is home to one of the four major world tennis events.
   Wimbledon

7. The running of the bulls takes place in this town in Spain each year.
   Pamplona

8. The Grand Ole Opry in this city hosts the Country Music Association awards.
   Nashville

9. The famous New Year's Day Rose Bowl Parade takes place here.
   Pasadena

10. In the 19th century, Texas fought a courageous battle at this location against the Republic of Mexico in their struggle for independence.
    Alamo

11. General Lee surrendered here to General Grant to end the Civil War.
    Appomattox Court House

12. The London Bridge was moved in 1971 from London, England, to this location in Arizona, USA.
    Lake Havasu

13. President Lincoln was shot at this theater in Washington, DC.
    Ford's Theatre

14. American colonists destroyed many crates of tea in this harbor.
    Boston

15. Mrs. O'Leary's cow kicked over a bucket to start a fire in this city.
    Chicago

16. The Pilgrims landed here in 1607 on the Mayflower.
    Plymouth Rock

FACILITATOR: *How many participants have visited these places? What other sites have they seen in these cities, states, or countries? Would they like to visit again? This would be a good opportunity to talk about car races and horse races. Who has been to either? Have they ever bet on a car or a horse? What about the running of the bulls? Is there anyone who would like to do that? Is the fame worth the risk? What do they think about moving a bridge all the way from London to Arizona?*

Some Like It Hot

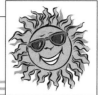

Whew, it's hot outside! Whether dry heat or humidity, nearly every state has its share of warm weather at some point during the year. The warm weather brings people out to celebrate Summer and enjoy swimming, sunbathing, and getting together with family and friends. Answer each question below (have a tall glass of lemonade on hand in case the heat is too much!).

1. Hot August Nights, a celebration of the 1950s culture of cars and rock and roll, is held each year in this city.

2. This is the warmest city in the United States, with more days each year over 89 degrees Fahrenheit than any other city.

3. This city in Arizona is the sunniest place on Earth, with the Sun shining 90% of the time.

4. December, January, February, and March are the warm Summer months in this part of the Earth.

5. A period of heat in early Fall is referred to as a what?

6. In 1995, an extreme heat wave in this U.S. city caused over 700 deaths.

7. Hot weather combined with little rainfall causes this phenomenon, which threatens crops, wildlife, and humans.

8. This warm city is known as the "Entertainment Capital of the World."

9. Every four years the Summer Olympics celebrate competition in over 25 warm-weather sports. Name three cities where they have been held.

10. Humidity can make warm weather downright uncomfortable. Name three U.S. states known for high humidity.

11. In tropical rainforest areas, these sudden, loud storms are a common occurrence.

12. These areas of sparse vegetation and little rainfall cover over one-third of Earth's surface.

13. Located in California, this national park is the hottest and driest in the United States.

14. This term describes the increase in Earth's temperature over the past 100 years and is the subject of much environmental study.

15. Invented in 1902 and readily available for homes and automobiles by the 1950s, the advent of this device made it possible to live comfortably in hot climates.

16. The Mojave Desert is an example of this type of desert, which is characterized by an elevation greater than 2,000 feet.

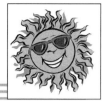

1. Hot August Nights, a celebration of the 1950s culture of cars and rock and roll, is held each year in this city.
   Reno

2. This is the warmest city in the United States, with more days each year over 89 degrees Fahrenheit than any other city.
   Phoenix

3. This city in Arizona is the sunniest place on Earth, with the Sun shining 90% of the time.
   Yuma

4. December, January, February, and March are the warm Summer months in this part of the Earth.
   south of the equator

5. A period of heat in early Fall is referred to as a what?
   Indian Summer

6. In 1995, an extreme heat wave in this U.S. city caused over 700 deaths.
   Chicago

7. Hot weather combined with little rainfall causes this phenomenon, which threatens crops, wildlife, and humans.
   drought

8. This warm city is known as the "Entertainment Capital of the World."
   Las Vegas

9. Every four years the Summer Olympics celebrate competition in over 25 warm-weather sports. Name three cities where they have been held.
   Los Angeles, Athens, Sydney, Barcelona, Seoul, Moscow, Montreal, Munich

10. Humidity can make warm weather downright uncomfortable. Name three U.S. states known for high humidity.
    Virginia, Louisiana, Florida, Georgia, North Carolina, South Carolina

11. In tropical rainforest areas, these sudden, loud storms are a common occurrence.
    thunderstorms

12. These areas of sparse vegetation and little rainfall cover over one-third of Earth's surface.
    desert

13. Located in California, this national park is the hottest and driest in the United States.
    Death Valley National Park

14. This term describes the increase in Earth's temperature over the past 100 years and is the subject of much environmental study.
    global warming

15. Invented in 1902 and readily available for homes and automobiles by the 1950s, the advent of this device made it possible to live comfortably in hot climates.
    air-conditioning

16. The Mojave Desert is an example of this type of desert, which is characterized by an elevation greater than 2,000 feet.
    high desert

FACILITATOR: The worksheet can be used to discuss with participants a variety of subjects related to warm weather. What was Summer like where you grew up? What did you do to cool off during Summer? Did your family have air-conditioning? Why or why not? Do you think that Earth is getting warmer? Do you prefer a warm climate or a cool climate? If possible, bring in maps so that the group can locate areas that are warm. Look for humid areas, dry areas, places where there are thunderstorms. You can also locate deserts and high deserts on a map.

Songs with Geographical Names in the Titles

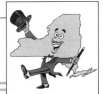

Many songs are written about special places—cities, states, rivers, mountains, and so forth. Can you name each of the songs described on the following two pages?

1. "East side, west side, all around the town" is the first line from this 1890s hit.

2. This Florida State song, written by Stephen Foster in 1851, takes place "way down" upon a river.

3. The rose from this song is "the sweetest rose of color." The song was popularized by Mitch Miller in the 1950s.

4. "From sea to shining sea," this patriotic song from the 1890s is often considered by many to be a more appropriate national anthem of the United States than the current one.

5. This song, made famous by Tony Bennett, refers to the "City by the Bay."

6. This song tells the story of traveling by train from New York City to this place in Tennessee.

7. Frank Sinatra sang this song about "that toddlin' town." It was his "kind of town."

8. This World War II song refers to the "bluebirds over" these, located on the English coastline.

9. This western ballad, also known as "Cowboy's Lament," was sung by Johnny Cash, Roy Rogers, and many other country singers. They "spied a young cowboy all wrapped in white linen / Wrapped in white linen as cold as the clay."

10. "Nothing could be finer than . . . " this Tin Pan Alley hit from the early 1900s.

11. In this song, Elvis Presley bids you to "Come with me / While the moon is on the sea" on this very colorful island.

12. Originally named "In Other Words," in this song Frank Sinatra yearns to "Fill my heart with song / Let me sing forever more."

13. It was written for the movie *Gold Diggers of 1935* and won the Academy Award for Best Original Song.

14. Saying good-bye to this large city in Italy is the topic of this song, one of Perry Como's most famous.

15. This George M. Cohan song was performed by James Cagney in the movie *Yankee Doodle Dandy*. "Remember me to Herald Square" is one of its famous lines.

16. This western ballad, popularized by Marty Robbins, refers to an "Out in the West Texas town" where "I fell in love with a Mexican girl."

17. This song was written about a city on the banks of Lake Michigan. "Not Louisiana, Paris, France, New York, or Rome, but . . . "

18. This jazz song, written in 1935, is about nighttime in a large city in Florida.

19. This popular Christmas carol is about a town where "The hopes and fears of all the years are met in thee tonight."

20. "Come and sit by my side if you love me" is a line sung by cowboys in this folk song often performed by The Sons of The Pioneers.

21. This song is the theme from a musical of the same name by Rodgers and Hammerstein. It includes the line "Ev'ry night my honey lamb and I sit alone and talk and watch a hawk makin' lazy circles in the sky."

22. This song, often performed by Patti Page, was about a friend who, while they were dancing, "stole my sweetheart from me."

23. This is the official state song of a midwestern state. Its chorus begins "Drifting with the current down a moonlit stream."

24. "It's a long way to go to see the sweetest girl I know." This very popular song, written about a place in Ireland, has been used as a theme song, as a wartime song, and as a marching song.

25. "We will dance the hoochie coochie / I will be your tootsie wootsie / If you will meet me in . . . ," is the theme song from a movie of the same name.

26. This theme song from a movie of the same name was popularized by Liza Minnelli and often serves as a theme song of this city. It is often played shortly after midnight on New Year's Eve in New York's Times Square.

27. "I'll be standing on the corner / On the corner of Twelfth Street and Vine" explains where the singer will be in this city.

28. This song from *South Pacific* is the name of a special fictional island that "may call you, any night, any day."

29. "I wish I was in the land of cotton" is the first line of this 19th-century folk song from the South.

30. This 1850s Stephen Foster song describes slave life on a plantation. It was originally called "Poor Uncle Tom, Good Night!" It is now a state song.

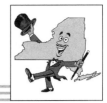

1. "East side, west side, all around the town" is the first line from this 1890s hit.
   "Sidewalks of New York"

2. This Florida State song, written by Stephen Foster in 1851, takes place "way down" upon a river.
   "Down Upon the Swanee River (Old Folks at Home)"

3. The rose from this song is "the sweetest rose of color." The song was popularized by Mitch Miller in the 1950s.
   "The Yellow Rose of Texas"

4. "From sea to shining sea," this patriotic song from the 1890s is often considered by many to be a more appropriate national anthem of the United States than the current one.
   "America the Beautiful"

5. This song, made famous by Tony Bennett, refers to the "City by the Bay."
   "I Left My Heart in San Francisco"

6. This song tells the story of traveling by train from New York City to this place in Tennessee.
   "Chattanooga Choo-Choo"

7. Frank Sinatra sang this song about "that toddlin' town." It was his "kind of town."
   "Chicago"

8. This World War II song refers to the "bluebirds over" these, located on the English coastline.
   "White Cliffs of Dover"

9. This western ballad, also known as "Cowboy's Lament," was sung by Johnny Cash, Roy Rogers, and many other country singers. They "spied a young cowboy all wrapped in white linen / Wrapped in white linen as cold as the clay."
   "Streets of Laredo"

10. "Nothing could be finer than . . . " this Tin Pan Alley hit from the early 1900s.
    "Carolina in the Morning"

11. In this song, Elvis Presley bids you to "Come with me / While the moon is on the sea" on this very colorful island.
    "Blue Hawaii"

12. Originally named "In Other Words," in this song Frank Sinatra yearns to "Fill my heart with song / Let me sing forever more."
    "Fly Me to the Moon"

13. "Come on along and listen to" is the first line of this song, one of Doris Day's most famous hits. It was written for the movie *Gold Diggers of 1935* and won the Academy Award for Best Original Song.
    "Lullaby of Broadway"

14. Saying good-bye to this large city in Italy is the topic of this song, one of Perry Como's most famous.
    "Arrivederci Roma"

15. This George M. Cohan song was performed by James Cagney in the movie *Yankee Doodle Dandy*. "Remember me to Herald Square" is one of its famous lines.
    "Give My Regards to Broadway"

16. This western ballad, popularized by Marty Robbins, refers to an "Out in the West Texas town" where "I fell in love with a Mexican girl."
    "El Paso"

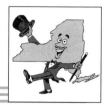

17. This song was written about a city on the banks of Lake Michigan. "Not Louisiana, Paris, France, New York, or Rome, but . . . "
"Gary, Indiana"

18. This jazz song, written in 1935, is about nighttime in a large city in Florida.
"Moon Over Miami"

19. This popular Christmas carol is about a town where "The hopes and fears of all the years are met in thee tonight."
"Oh Little Town of Bethlehem"

20. "Come and sit by my side if you love me" is a line sung by cowboys in this folk song often performed by The Sons of The Pioneers.
"Red River Valley"

21. This song is the theme from a musical of the same name by Rodgers and Hammerstein. It includes the line "Ev'ry night my honey lamb and I sit alone and talk and watch a hawk makin' lazy circles in the sky."
"Oklahoma"

22. This song, often performed by Patti Page, was about a friend who, while they were dancing, "stole my sweetheart from me."
"Tennessee Waltz"

23. This is the official state song of a midwestern state. Its chorus begins "Drifting with the current down a moonlit stream."
"Beautiful Ohio"

24. "It's a long way to go to see the sweetest girl I know." This very popular song, written about a place in Ireland, has been used as a theme song, as a wartime song, and as a marching song.
"It's a Long Way to Tiperrary"

25. "We will dance the hoochie coochie / I will be your tootsie wootsie / If you will meet me in . . . ," is the theme song from a movie of the same name.
"Meet Me in St. Louis, Louis"

26. This theme song from a movie of the same name was popularized by Liza Minnelli and often serves as a theme song of this city. It is often played shortly after midnight on New Year's Eve in New York's Times Square.
"New York, New York"

27. "I'll be standing on the corner / On the corner of Twelfth Street and Vine" explains where the singer will be in this city.
"Kansas City"

28. This song from *South Pacific* is the name of a special fictional island that "may call you, any night, any day."
"Bali Ha'i"

29. "I wish I was in the land of cotton" is the first line of this 19th-century folk song from the South.
"Dixie"

30. This 1850s Stephen Foster song describes slave life on a plantation. It was originally called "Poor Uncle Tom, Good Night!" It is now a state song.
"My Old Kentucky Home"

FACILITATOR: This activity is sure to bring lots of singing to the group. You might want to copy the words to some or all of these songs so that the group can sing an entire song. Ask for favorites. Who do they know that sang each song? Which ones were songs from movies? When and where did they first learn the lyrics to any of the songs? Have they seen any singers perform any of the songs?

Space and Beyond

Humankind has had a fascination with flight for hundreds of years, since before China discovered in 400 BC that kites could fly. Advances continue and, as they say, "the sky's the limit." Who knows what type of flight will come next? The following facts all pertain to flight. Can you name each item?

1. A tire and rubber company uses this airship to advertise.

2. Clark Kent changes clothes in a telephone booth to become this.

3. This German zeppelin, a very large type of aircraft, caught fire in New Jersey in 1937. It was named after the German president at the time.

4. How many major airlines can you name?

5. These pilots fly a certain color plane and act as goodwill ambassadors for the U.S. Navy and Marine Corps, often performing in air shows.

6. This American general was the first pilot to travel faster than the speed of sound.

7. In 1927, Charles Lindbergh flew the first trans-Atlantic nonstop flight in this plane from Long Island, New York, to Paris, France.

8. She was the first female to receive the Distinguished Flying Cross for her solo flight across the Atlantic.

9. Another name for this unpowered aircraft that "soars" through the air is a sailplane.

10. This World War I ace fighter pilot's 26 "aerial victories" won him a multitude of medals.

11. This Jules Verne movie chronicles a trip around the globe.

12. This company is the largest global aircraft manufacturer. Among their current plans are the 747 and 787.

13. Someone who caters to the needs of passengers on commercial airlines is called what?

14. This billionaire eccentric recluse produced and flew his own plane in 1947, named the Spruce Goose.

15. How many objects can you name that can be flown?

16. This American aviator flew from Long Beach, California, to New York and was supposed to return to Long Beach, but instead flew to Ireland. He claimed that his unauthorized flight was due to "navigational error"!

1. A tire and rubber company uses this airship to advertise.
   Goodyear Blimp

2. Clark Kent changes clothes in a telephone booth to become this.
   Superman

3. This German zeppelin, a very large type of aircraft, caught fire in New Jersey in 1937. It was named after the German president at the time.
   Hindenburg

4. How many major airlines can you name?
   Air Canada, Air France, Alaska, All Nippon (Japan), American, British Airways, Continental, Delta, Iberia, Japan Airlines, KLM, Korean Air, Lufthansa, Northwest, Pan-Am, Qantas, Southwest, TWA, United, US Airways

5. These pilots fly a certain color plane and act as goodwill ambassadors for the U.S. Navy and Marine Corps, often performing in air shows.
   Blue Angels

6. This American general was the first pilot to travel faster than the speed of sound.
   Chuck Yeager

7. In 1927, Charles Lindbergh flew the first trans-Atlantic nonstop flight in this plane from Long Island, New York, to Paris, France.
   Spirit of St. Louis

8. She was the first female to receive the Distinguished Flying Cross for her solo flight across the Atlantic.
   Amelia Earhart

9. Another name for this unpowered aircraft that "soars" through the air is a sailplane.
   glider

10. This World War I ace fighter pilot's 26 "aerial victories" won him a multitude of medals.
    Edward Rickenbacker

11. This Jules Verne movie chronicles a trip around the globe.
    Around the World in 80 Days

12. This company is the largest global aircraft manufacturer. Among their current plans are the 747 and 787.
    Boeing

13. Someone who caters to the needs of passengers on commercial airlines is called what?
    Flight attendant, stewardess, steward

14. This billionaire eccentric recluse produced and flew his own plane in 1947, named the Spruce Goose.
    Howard Hughes

15. How many objects can you name that can be flown?
    kite, helicopter, blimp, hot air balloon, dirigible, parasail

16. This American aviator flew from Long Beach, California, to New York and was supposed to return to Long Beach, but instead flew to Ireland. He claimed that his unauthorized flight was due to "navigational error"!
    Douglas "Wrong-Way" Corrigan

FACILITATOR: *Depending on the interests of the group, this activity could be steered in a number of different directions. When and where was their first trip on a plane? Have they ever been on a small plane? Which airline do they like best? How much do they think a ticket to certain places would cost. You might want to bring in some ads from the travel section of a magazine or newspaper to share with participants.*

This Is the Place

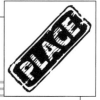

As several of the activities in this section show, there are places of interest all over the world. The term *place* has its "place" in everyday conversation. For this worksheet, read the description and provide the answer. (Hint: each answer has the word *place* in it.)

1. A person who feels as though he or she does not fit in might feel this way.

2. A plate, silverware, and napkin make up a what?

3. A person who will be very successful is going to what?

4. A very popular hangout is called the what?

5. This type of kick is used in rugby football.

6. In gambling, to wager is to what?

7. In school, college-level courses that are offered at high school are called what?

8. If you have friends with power and influence, it is said that you have friends in what?

9. To bring an arrogant or overconfident person down is to what?

10. Many religious buildings are called what?

11. In football, the person responsible for kicking field goals, extra points, and kickoffs is called the what?

12. In college, the service that assists students with finding a job is called a what?

13. To substitute one thing for another is to have it _____ the other.

14. Another way to describe something that is everywhere is what?

15. To call someone on the telephone is to what?

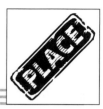

1. A person who feels as though he or she does not fit in might feel this way.
   out of place

2. A plate, silverware, and napkin make up a what?
   place setting

3. A person who will be very successful is going to what?
   go places

4. A very popular hangout is called the what?
   place to be

5. This type of kick is used in rugby football.
   placekick

6. In gambling, to wager is to what?
   place a bet

7. In school, college-level courses that are offered at high school are called what?
   advanced placement

8. If you have friends with power and influence, it is said that you have friends in what?
   high places

9. To bring an arrogant or overconfident person down is to what?
   put a person in his or her place

10. Many religious buildings are called what?
    place of worship

11. In football, the person responsible for kicking field goals, extra points, and kickoffs is called the what?
    placekicker

12. In college, the service that assists students with finding a job is called a what?
    placement office

13. To substitute one thing for another is to have it _____ the other.
    in place of

14. Another way to describe something that is everywhere is what?
    all over the place

15. To call someone on the telephone is to what?
    place a call

FACILITATOR: *This worksheet can be used to encourage conversation about several topics. Ask participants the following questions: How do you think these words and phrases came about? How often are these used in everyday talk? Do people in the group have a favorite place they have visited or lived? What makes something stand out as a special place?*

The West Coast

Horace Greeley once said, "Go west, young man, go west." Over the last two hundred years, people have been doing just that. They have headed west for a variety of reasons. Millions have ended up on the West Coast. The following activity contains many facts about the western coastal states. How many of these facts are familiar to you?

1. The West Coast borders which ocean?

2. There are five states that border this ocean. Can you name them?

3. The Space Needle for the 1962 World's Fair was built in this city.

4. The Golden Gate Bridge, one of the most famous in the world, is located in this "City by the Bay."

5. The first overland expedition to the West Coast was led by these two men.

6. This city is known as "The City of Roses."

7. This state is geographically the largest in the United States.

8. The San Andreas fault runs through northwestern California and is the source of many of these.

9. This state is the only state completely surrounded by water.

10. This state hosts the annual Iditarod sled dog race.

11. This is the only U.S. capital that is accessible only by sea or air.

12. This food is a staple of the Big Island and is made from taro.

13. These two states were admitted to the Union in 1959.

14. Can you name three West Coast professional baseball teams?

15. The most populous state in the United States is on the West Coast. Which one is it?

16. This West Coast state is the only one named after a president.

17. The Columbia River and Crater Lake are two famous bodies of water located in this state.

18. Cable cars are one of this city's landmarks.

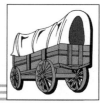

1. The West Coast borders which ocean?
   Pacific

2. There are five states that border this ocean. Can you name them?
   Alaska, California, Hawaii, Oregon, Washington

3. The Space Needle for the 1962 World's Fair was built in this city.
   Seattle

4. The Golden Gate Bridge, one of the most famous in the world, is located in this "City by the Bay."
   San Francisco

5. The first overland expedition to the West Coast was led by these two men.
   Meriwether Lewis and William Clark

6. This city is known as "The City of Roses."
   Portland

7. This state is geographically the largest in the United States.
   Alaska

8. The San Andreas fault runs through northwestern California and is the source of many of these.
   earthquakes

9. This state is the only state completely surrounded by water.
   Hawaii

10. This state hosts the annual Iditarod sled dog race.
    Alaska

11. This is the only U.S. capital that is accessible only by sea or air.
    Juneau

12. This food is a staple of the Big Island and is made from taro.
    poi

13. These two states were admitted to the Union in 1959.
    Alaska and Hawaii

14. Can you name three West Coast professional baseball teams?
    Anaheim Angels, L.A. Dodgers, Oakland Athletics, San Diego Padres, San Francisco Giants, Seattle Mariners

15. The most populous state in the United States is on the West Coast. Which one is it?
    California (with over 36 million residents)

16. This West Coast state is the only one named after a president.
    Washington

17. The Columbia River and Crater Lake are two famous bodies of water located in this state.
    Oregon

18. Cable cars are one of this city's landmarks.
    San Francisco

FACILITATOR: *As with all activities that involve locations, a map would be useful. Ask how many of these states each person has visited. Which is his or her favorite and why? What other facts do participants know about the West Coast? Why do they think that people pushed west instead of staying in the east? What made it so enticing? Do they think life on the West Coast is much different than life on the East Coast?*

Which Continent Is It?

Africa, Antarctica, Asia, Australia, Europe, North America, and South America are the seven continents on Earth. They vary greatly in size, population, geography, culture, economy, and just about every other characteristic. Each of the following facts pertains to one of these continents. How many can you name?

1. Which is the largest continent in size?

2. Which is the smallest continent in size?

3. Which continent is home to the most number of people?

4. Which continent is home to the fewest number of people?

5. Which two continents are divided by the Ural Mountains?

6. To which continent did the British send their prisoners in the 17th and 18th centuries?

7. Which continent has the largest river system (not the longest)?

8. Which continent is home to the southernmost city (Punta Arenas)?

9. Which continent has the highest point on Earth?

10. Which continent contains most of the world's gold and diamonds?

11. Which continent is home to the world's largest freshwater lake?

12. Which is the only continent on which tigers are found?

13. Which continent has more sheep than people?

14. Which continent has the lowest mean elevation?

15. To which continent does Central America belong?

16. This continent has the largest economy on Earth.

17. The following cities are the largest in which continent (as of 2008)?
    a. New York City
    b. Tokyo
    c. Lagos
    d. Moscow
    e. São Paulo
    f. Sydney

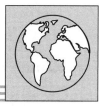

1. Which is the largest continent in size?
    Asia

2. Which is the smallest continent in size?
    Australia

3. Which continent is home to the most number of people?
    Asia

4. Which continent is home to the fewest number of people?
    Antarctica (population 0)

5. Which two continents are divided by the Ural Mountains?
    Asia and Europe

6. To which continent did the British send their prisoners in the 17th and 18th centuries?
    Australia

7. Which continent has the largest river system (not the longest)?
    South America (Amazon)

8. Which continent is home to the southernmost city (Punta Arenas)?
    South America

9. Which continent has the highest point on Earth?
    Asia with Mt. Everest (29,000 feet)

10. Which continent contains most of the world's gold and diamonds?
    Africa

11. Which continent is home to the world's largest freshwater lake?
    North America (Superior)

12. Which is the only continent on which tigers are found?
    Asia

13. Which continent has more sheep than people?
    Australia

14. Which continent has the lowest mean elevation?
    Antarctica

15. To which continent does Central America belong?
    North America

16. This continent has the largest economy on Earth.
    Europe

17. The following cities are the largest in which continent (as of 2008)?
    a. **New York City**   **North America**
    b. **Tokyo**   **Asia**
    c. **Lagos**   **Africa (Nigeria)**
    d. **Moscow**   **Europe**
    e. **São Paulo**   **South America (Brazil)**
    f. **Sydney**   **Australia**

FACILITATOR: *This is a great activity for all people, no matter where in the world they are from. Be sure and use a map to locate the answers. Ask participants what they know about each continent. How many have they been to? Which would they like to visit? What would they like to see on their visit? You might want to discuss food, religion, government, music, languages, and so forth about each continent. How many countries can they name from each continent?*

Which Country Is It?

Each country in the world is known for many things—some for food, some for politics, some for famous people, some for infamous people, some for their geography. Can you name the country to which the following facts refer? If you'd like a little help, the countries are listed at the bottom of this page.

1. Rhine River / Berlin Wall / Albert Einstein / hofbrau and beer

2. Houses of Parliament / Big Ben / Thames River / Stonehenge / Winchester Cathedral

3. Edinburgh Castle / bagpipes / kilts / St. Andrews Eden golf course / Loch Ness Monster

4. Eiffel Tower / Louvre / Bordeaux / champagne / Champs Elysses / most visited country in the world / Marie Antoinette

5. second-largest country in the world / ten provinces / St. Lawrence River / British commonwealth

6. largest country in the world / Red Square / Leningrad / Bolshevik Revolution / first astronaut to circle Earth

7. pasta / Tuscany / Colosseum / gondolas / Isle of Capri / Michelangelo

8. Acropolis / Parthenon / first Olympics / Athens

9. neutral / Zurich / Alps / chocolate / clocks

10. waltz / Mozart / Sigmund Freud / Vienna

11. Aztecs / Cinco de Mayo / Acapulco / Hidalgo / Mayan ruins / most populous Spanish-speaking country in the world

12. Eire / Gaelic football and hurling / Blarney Stone

13. Mandarin / Ming Dynasty / Confucius / New Year / Buddhism

14. Great Barrier Reef / Sydney Opera House / down under / kangaroos

15. Land of the Midnight Sun / over 3,000 islands / Mount Fuji / samurai / sumo wrestling / Toyota

16. Great Pyramids at Giza / Sphinx / Nile River / Anwar Sadat / muslim

17. Andes / Santiago / end of Pan American Highway / Pablo Neruda / Atacama Desert / Easter Island / long and narrow country

18. South Asia / second-most populated country in the world / Taj Mahal / its capital New Delhi / Gandhi

Choices: Australia, Austria, Canada, Chile, China, Egypt, England, France, Germany, Greece, India, Ireland, Italy, Japan, Mexico, Russia, Scotland, Switzerland

Which Country Is It? ANSWER SHEET

1. Rhine River / Berlin Wall / Albert Einstein / hofbrau and beer
   Germany
2. Houses of Parliament / Big Ben / Thames River / Stonehenge / Winchester Cathedral
   England
3. Edinburgh Castle / bagpipes / kilts / St. Andrews Eden golf course / Loch Ness Monster
   Scotland
4. Eiffel Tower / Louvre / Bordeaux / champagne / Champs Elysses / most visited country in the world / Marie Antoinette
   France
5. second-largest country in the world / ten provinces / St. Lawrence River / British commonwealth
   Canada
6. largest country in the world / Red Square / Leningrad / Bolshevik Revolution / first astronaut to circle Earth
   Russia
7. pasta / Tuscany / Colosseum / gondolas / Isle of Capri / Michelangelo
   Italy
8. Acropolis / Parthenon / first Olympics / Athens
   Greece
9. neutral / Zurich / Alps / chocolate / clocks
   Switzerland
10. waltz / Mozart / Sigmund Freud / Vienna
    Austria
11. Aztecs / Cinco de Mayo / Acapulco / Hidalgo / Mayan ruins / most populous Spanish-speaking country in the world
    Mexico
12. Eire / Gaelic football and hurling / Blarney Stone
    Ireland
13. Mandarin / Ming Dynasty / Confucius / New Year / Buddhism
    China
14. Great Barrier Reef / Sydney Opera House / down under / kangaroos
    Australia
15. Land of the Midnight Sun / over 3,000 islands / Mount Fuji / samurai / sumo wrestling / Toyota
    Japan
16. Great Pyramids at Giza / Sphinx / Nile River / Anwar Sadat / muslim
    Egypt
17. Andes / Santiago / end of Pan American Highway / Pablo Neruda / Atacama Desert / Easter Island / long and narrow country
    Chile
18. South Asia / second-most populated country in the world / Taj Mahal / its capital New Delhi / Gandhi
    India

FACILITATOR: *Be sure and use a map when completing this activity. Ask if participants can name any additional clues that might be given for these countries. How many of these countries have they visited? Which sites have they seen? Which other countries could be added to this list?*

Which State Is It?

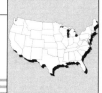

All 50 U.S. states are famous for a number of reasons—some good, some bad! Some of the reasons may be familiar to you, and others may be a surprise. The facts on the following three pages all pertain to one of each of the states. Can you guess each state? If you would like a list of all 50 states to help you, one is included on the last page of this activity.

1. Golden Gate Bridge / discovery of gold in 1848 / redwoods

2. Big Apple / Statue of Liberty / Yankees / Erie Canal / Wall Street

3. largest state / only state capital unreachable by car / oil pipeline / Aleutian Islands / Last Frontier / Mt. McKinley

4. Space Needle / home of Starbucks Coffee / Seahawks / Mt. Rainier / Mt. St. Helens

5. Grand Canyon / cactus / Hoover Dam / gunfight at O.K. Corral / Geronimo

6. Everglades / Kennedy Space Center / Ponce de Leon / St. Augustine

7. Louis Armstrong / cajun food / only state capital below sea level / Mardi Gras

8. smallest state / Providence / Newport

9. Big Sky country / Custer's Last Stand / Glacier National Park

10. Least populated state / first state to give women right to vote / Yellowstone National Park

11. Brigham Young / Great Salt Lake / hosted 2002 Winter Olympics / Zion National Park

12. Highest mean elevation of any state / Pike's Peak / Mile High City / Coors beer / Rocky Mountain National Park / Mesa Verde

13. volcanoes / poi / 50th state / settled by Polynesians

14. automakers / Wolverines / borders four of five Great Lakes

15. German influence / Brewers / cheese / Green Bay

16. Booker T. Washington / George Washington Carver / 1965 freedom march / Civil Rights movement / Rosa Parks

17. Yale University / insurance capital / richest state

18. Portsmouth / its primary election considered national forecaster / Granite State

19. first state to ratify Constitution / Dover / Diamond State

20. Carlsbad Caverns / Billy the Kid / Los Alamos

21. Stone Mountain / home of Coca-Cola / Peach State / Jimmy Carter

22. Roanoke Island / Kitty Hawk / Blue Ridge National Parkway

23. Snake River / Gem State / potatoes

24. Ozarks / Bill Clinton / Little Rock

25. Hoosiers / famous car race ("500") / Notre Dame

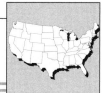

26. blue crabs / Chesapeake Bay / Annapolis / Orioles / Fort McHenry

27. Hawkeye State / biggest corn producer / Herbert Hoover

28. Daniel Boone / tobacco / whiskey / Louisville / Churchill Downs

29. Lincoln / Windy City / Cubs / White Sox

30. Atlantic City / Princeton University / Garden State / Frank Sinatra

31. lobster / pine trees / Acadia National Park

32. John Brown / Harper's Ferry / Mountain State / Appalachian Mountains

33. Vikings / Twin Cities / Land of 10,000 Lakes

34. largest river / cotton / birthplace of Elvis

35. wheat fields / Fort Leavenworth / Wizard of Oz

36. Mark Twain / Harry Truman / Show Me State

37. ten-gallon hats / oil / Rangers / Alamo / Sam Houston

38. Cornhuskers / Gerald Ford / cottonwood trees

39. driest state / Comstock Lode / marriage capital of the U.S. / gambling

40. Jamestown / birthplace of eight presidents / Mt. Vernon / Shenandoah National Park

41. Buckeyes / Pro Football Hall of Fame / birthplace of seven presidents

42. clam chowder / Harvard / Plymouth Colony / Tea Party / Cape Cod

43. land rush / Will Rogers / Cowboy Hall of Fame / panhandle / Sooners

44. City of Roses / Crater Lake / Pacific Northwest / mouth of Columbia River

45. Dutch / William Penn / Declaration of Independence / Liberty Bell / Gettysburg / Valley Forge

46. most rural of all states / Rough Riders / Sioux Indians

47. plantations / Fort Sumter / first state to secede from Union / Charleston

48. Graceland / Great Smokey Mountains / Davy Crockett

49. maple syrup / Green Mountain Boys / Calvin Coolidge / Ethan Allen

50. Mt. Rushmore / Black Hills / Badlands National Park

The 50 states: Alabama, Alaska, Arizona, Arkansas, California, Colorado, Connecticut, Delaware, Florida, Georgia, Hawaii, Idaho, Iowa, Illinois, Indiana, Kansas, Kentucky, Louisiana, Maine, Maryland, Massachusetts, Michigan, Minnesota, Mississippi, Missouri, Montana, Nebraska, Nevada, New Hampshire, New Jersey, New Mexico, New York, North Carolina, North Dakota, Ohio, Oklahoma, Oregon, Pennsylvania, Rhode Island, South Carolina, South Dakota, Tennessee, Texas, Utah, Vermont, Virginia, Washington, West Virginia, Wisconsin, Wyoming

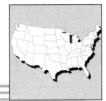

1. Golden Gate Bridge / discovery of gold in 1848 / redwoods
   California

2. Big Apple / Statue of Liberty / Yankees / Erie Canal / Wall Street
   New York

3. largest state / only state capital unreachable by car / oil pipeline / Aleutian Islands / Last Frontier / Mt. McKinley
   Alaska

4. Space Needle / home of Starbucks Coffee / Seahawks / Mt. Rainier / Mt. St. Helens
   Washington

5. Grand Canyon / cactus / Hoover Dam / gunfight at O.K. Corral / Geronimo
   Arizona

6. Everglades / Kennedy Space Center / Ponce de Leon / St. Augustine
   Florida

7. Louis Armstrong / cajun food / only state capital below sea level / Mardi Gras
   Louisiana

8. smallest state / Providence / Newport
   Rhode Island

9. Big Sky country / Custer's Last Stand / Glacier National Park
   Montana

10. Least populated state / first state to give women right to vote / Yellowstone National Park
    Wyoming

11. Brigham Young / Great Salt Lake / hosted 2002 Winter Olympics / Zion National Park
    Utah

12. Highest mean elevation of any state / Pike's Peak / Mile High City / Coors beer / Rocky Mountain National Park / Mesa Verde
    Colorado

13. volcanoes / poi / 50th state / settled by Polynesians
    Hawaii

14. automakers / Wolverines / borders four of five Great Lakes
    Michigan

15. German influence / Brewers / cheese / Green Bay
    Wisconsin

16. Booker T. Washington / George Washington Carver / 1965 freedom march / Civil Rights movement / Rosa Parks
    Alabama

17. Yale University / insurance capital / richest state
    Connecticut

18. Portsmouth / its primary election considered national forecaster / Granite State
    New Hampshire

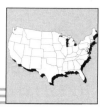

Which State Is It? ANSWER SHEET (CONTINUED)

19. first state to ratify Constitution / Dover / Diamond State
    Delaware

20. Carlsbad Caverns / Billy the Kid / Los Alamos
    New Mexico

21. Stone Mountain / home of Coca-Cola / Peach State / Jimmy Carter
    Georgia

22. Roanoke Island / Kitty Hawk / Blue Ridge National Parkway
    North Carolina

23. Snake River / Gem State / potatoes
    Idaho

24. Ozarks / Bill Clinton / Little Rock
    Arkansas

25. Hoosiers / famous car race ("500") / Notre Dame
    Indiana

26. blue crabs / Chesapeake Bay / Annapolis / Orioles / Fort McHenry
    Maryland

27. Hawkeye State / biggest corn producer / Herbert Hoover
    Iowa

28. Daniel Boone / tobacco / whiskey / Louisville / Churchill Downs
    Kentucky

29. Lincoln / Windy City / Cubs / White Sox
    Illinois

30. Atlantic City / Princeton University / Garden State / Frank Sinatra
    New Jersey

31. lobster / pine trees / Acadia National Park
    Maine

32. John Brown / Harper's Ferry / Mountain State / Appalachian Mountains
    West Virginia

33. Vikings / Twin Cities / Land of 10,000 Lakes
    Minnesota

34. largest river / cotton / birthplace of Elvis
    Mississippi

35. wheat fields / Fort Leavenworth / Wizard of Oz
    Kansas

36. Mark Twain / Harry Truman / Show Me State
    Missouri

37. ten-gallon hats / oil / Rangers / Alamo / Sam Houston
    Texas

38. Cornhuskers / Gerald Ford / cottonwood trees
    Nebraska

Strengthen Your Mind, Volume Two by Einberger & Sellick. Copyright © 2008 by Health Professions Press, Inc.

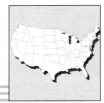

39. driest state / Comstock Lode / marriage capital of the U.S. / gambling
    Nevada

40. Jamestown / birthplace of eight presidents / Mt. Vernon / Shenandoah National Park
    Virginia

41. Buckeyes / Pro Football Hall of Fame / birthplace of seven presidents
    Ohio

42. clam chowder / Harvard / Plymouth Colony / Tea Party / Cape Cod
    Massachusetts

43. land rush / Will Rogers / Cowboy Hall of Fame / panhandle / Sooners
    Oklahoma

44. City of Roses / Crater Lake / Pacific Northwest / mouth of Columbia River
    Oregon

45. Dutch / William Penn / Declaration of Independence / Liberty Bell / Gettysburg / Valley Forge
    Pennsylvania

46. most rural of all states / Rough Riders / Sioux Indians
    North Dakota

47. plantations / Fort Sumter / first state to secede from Union / Charleston
    South Carolina

48. Graceland / Great Smokey Mountains / Davy Crockett
    Tennessee

49. maple syrup / Green Mountain Boys / Calvin Coolidge / Ethan Allen
    Vermont

50. Mt. Rushmore / Black Hills / Badlands National Park
    South Dakota

FACILITATOR: *This activity is sure to raise much interest as participants recall states where they were born, where they lived throughout their lives, and where they visited for various reasons. Be sure to use a map when completing this activity. Depending on the group, you may try giving only one clue at a time to see if they can answer with less than three clues. Ask people where they were born. Discuss the importance and relevance of the various clues. Can they think of other clues that could be given for each state? How many states have they visited? Which is their favorite? How many capitals can they name? Can they name famous people from any of the states? For sports fans, try asking which teams are from each state. For nature buffs, ask which states have famous national or state parks. A great activity to accompany these questions would be to give everyone a blank U.S. map and have them fill in as many states as possible. To take this even further, have them write in the state capitals.*

Things

We are surrounded by things in everyday life. So many, in fact, that there are endless mentally stimulating topics that are related to things. The dictionary defines the word *thing* as "an unspecified material, object, person, or animal." In this section of the book, you will find worksheets with a variety of subjects. For some you may need to take a look at yourself (*Where on the Human Body Is . . . ?*), and for others you may need to think back to some of the clothing you wore in past years (*Passing Fads*). Regardless of the order in which you do the worksheets, there is no doubt you will enjoy challenging your mind with the variety of activities in this section.

All About Arches

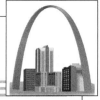

The arch is a historical shape that is used in architecture all over the world. Evidence of the first arch dates back to ancient Rome. Today we find arches everywhere, from restaurant symbols to our own bodies. Read the description of the arch on the left and match it with the answer on the right.

_____ 1. This national park located in Utah is home to over 2,000 natural sandstone arches.

_____ 2. This arch, also called the Jefferson National Expansion Memorial, is located in St. Louis, Missouri.

_____ 3. These arches are found all over the world and are the symbol of McDonald's restaurants.

_____ 4. In a masonry arch, or an arch made with bricks or stone, there is always a stone that marks the top of the arch. What is this stone called?

_____ 5. A person who is your sworn enemy or competition is called a what?

_____ 6. The curve on the bottom of a foot is called what?

_____ 7. The New River Gorge Bridge in West Virginia is an example of this type of bridge.

_____ 8. Located in Arches National Park, this famous arch became the symbol for the state of Utah.

_____ 9. A passage under an arch or a group of arches is called a what?

_____ 10. This famous arch in Paris was built in the 1800s to honor soldiers who fought for France and is the location of the tomb of the unknown soldier.

_____ 11. In 1828, this London arch was originally designed as the entryway to Buckingham Palace but now resides in Hyde Park.

_____ 12. In the Christian Church, the head unit of a group of churches is called a what?

_____ 13. A series of arches used in building ancient aqueducts, such as the Roman aqueducts, is called what?

_____ 14. In architecture, an arch that has been filled in so that nothing can pass beneath it is called a what?

_____ 15. Located in Hartford, New Hampshire, this arch was built in 1886 to honor Hartford citizens who served in the Civil War.

_____ 16. Crossing the U.S. border from California into Mexico you will find this arch, a namesake for a popular border city.

_____ 17. In religion, an angel who receives the highest ranking or level is called a what?

a. Arc de Triomphe

b. arch of the foot

c. blind arch

d. arch bridge

e. Arches National Park

f. archdiocese

g. golden arches

h. Soldiers and Sailors Arch

i. Gateway Arch

j. keystone (or capstone)

k. Delicate Arch

l. arcades

m. Tijuana Arch

n. archway

o. archangel

p. arch rival

q. Marble Arch

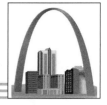

1. This national park located in Utah is home to over 2,000 natural sandstone arches.

   e. **Arches National Park**

2. This arch, also called the Jefferson National Expansion Memorial, is located in St. Louis, Missouri.

   i. **Gateway Arch**

3. These arches are found all over the world and are the symbol of McDonald's restaurants.

   g. **golden arches**

4. In a masonry arch, or an arch made with bricks or stone, there is always a stone that marks the top of the arch. What is this stone called?

   j. **keystone (or capstone)**

5. A person who is your sworn enemy or competition is called a what?

   p. **arch rival**

6. The curve on the bottom of a foot is called what?

   b. **arch of the foot**

7. The New River Gorge Bridge in West Virginia is an example of this type of bridge.

   d. **arch bridge**

8. Located in Arches National Park, this famous arch became the symbol for the state of Utah.

   k. **Delicate Arch**

9. A passage under an arch or a group of arches is called a what?

   n. **archway**

10. This famous arch in Paris was built in the 1800s to honor soldiers who fought for France and is the location of the tomb of the unknown soldier.

   j. **Arc de Triomphe**

11. In 1828, this London arch was originally designed as the entryway to Buckingham Palace but now resides in Hyde Park.

   q. **Marble Arch**

12. In the Christian Church, the head unit of a group of churches is called a what?

   f. **archdiocese**

13. A series of arches used in building ancient aqueducts, such as the Roman aqueducts, is called what?

   l. **arcades**

14. In architecture, an arch that has been filled in so that nothing can pass beneath it is called a what?

   c. **blind arch**

15. Located in Hartford, New Hampshire, this arch was built in 1886 to honor Hartford citizens who served in the Civil War.

   h. **Soldiers and Sailors Arch**

16. Crossing the U.S. border from California into Mexico you will find this arch, a namesake for a popular border city.

   m. **Tijuana Arch**

17. In religion, an angel who receives the highest ranking or level is called a what?

   o. **archangel**

FACILITATOR: *Use a map when discussing the arches that are landmarks. How many participants have visited these arches? What other purposes do arches serve in architecture? Other than the arch of the foot, are there other areas of the body that have an arch? What type of arches do you see around your town? What are some other important shapes in architecture?*

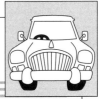

All-American Things

A–Z lists are a wonderful way to give the brain a mental workout! For this list, think of at least one all-American "thing" for each letter of the alphabet. For example, "apple pie" could be considered all American, as could "amendments."

A

B

C

D

E

F

G

H

I

J

K

L

M

N

O

P

Q

R

S

T

U

V

W

X

Y

Z

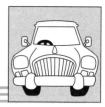

A   amendments / apple pie / Air Force

B   Bill of Rights / baseball / Buick

C   Constitution / Chevrolet / Civil War / Confederates

D   Declaration of Independence / democrats / democracy

E   executive branch / Edsel / entrepreneurship

F   flag / Fourth of July / FBI

G   Grand Old Flag / gold rush / General Motors

H   House of Representatives / hot dogs / Halloween

I   Indy 500 / Industrial Revolution / Independence Day

J   judicial system / jello / jury

K   Kentucky Derby / kick the can / Korean War

L   legislature / Labor Day / Liberty Bell

M   Mayflower / McDonald's / Marines

N   Niña / NASCAR / Navy

O   Old Glory / oath of office / oval office

P   primaries / president / Pilgrims / Pentagon

Q   the quarter / quiz shows / quill pen

R   republicans / red, white, and blue / Revolutionary War

S   Senate / stars and stripes / Santa Maria / Star Spangled Banner

T   thirteen colonies / Thanksgiving / trick or treating

U   Uncle Sam / Union Army / "United We Stand"

V   voting / Veterans Day / Vietnam War

W   Washington, DC / World War I / World War II / White House

X   Xmas / Xerox

Y   yellow ribbon / Yankees / Yellowstone National Park

Z   Zion National Park / ZIP code

FACILITATOR: *Encourage the group to think about all types of things that are all-American—foods, facets of political life, pastimes, and so forth. After the group is done, you can narrow the topic and ask them to make an A–Z list of just American foods or hobbies. For discussion, ask the group what makes something all-American? Of the things on the list, which make a participant the most proud to be an American?*

Animal Facts

There are millions of species of animals in the world, from the smallest, which can only be seen under a microscope, to the largest, which lives in the ocean. Can you name the animals described below?

1. This sleek animal is the fastest on land and is able to reach speeds of approximately 70 miles per hour for a short distance.

2. There are two kinds of this animal. The one from Africa is taller and has larger ears than the one from India.

3. The young of this mammal are called *joeys* and are the size of a bumblebee when born.

4. These social animals are the closest relatives to humans, are one of four types of great apes, and can be found in 21 African countries.

5. This nocturnal mammal is the only marsupial native to North America. It carries its young in a pouch for about two and half months after birth. Often when danger appears, this animal will fall to its side and appear to be dead.

6. This animal, which is not really a bear (although its name includes *bear*), can survive on a diet of eucalyptus leaves.

7. In this family, females are called *sows* and males *boars*. Although we hear otherwise, they would rather stay clean if given the chance.

8. This animal's height is measured in "hands." One hand equals about 4 inches. Many wear "shoes" on their feet for protection.

9. This large mammal can spend its whole life on the ice without ever setting foot on land. It feeds on a diet of meat, primarily seals.

10. This animal is the largest animal in existence, lives in the ocean, and is surrounded by a layer of fat called *blubber*. The largest ever recorded was 32 feet long and weighed 22,000 pounds!

11. This is the only mammal that can fly. They are nocturnal and are not "blind," as some believe they are.

12. This is the tallest animal in the world, measuring 6 feet when born. It often spreads its legs apart to drink, since its neck is too short to reach the ground otherwise.

13. These animals can spit a distance of 10 feet or more and are members of the camel family. They have been domesticated for thousands of years and are often used as pack animals.

14. This animal's roar can be heard up to 5 miles away. It lives mostly on the plains of Africa and generally in "prides."

15. This "sly" animal's most common species is red, although others include gray, arctic, kit and fennec. It is a solitary animal and hunts mostly at night. Its baby is called a *kit*.

16. This nocturnal animal often invades garbage cans. We often say that they look like "bandits" due to the area around their eyes being a little darker than the rest of their coloring.

Animal Facts ANSWER SHEET

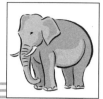

1. This sleek animal is the fastest on land and is able to reach speeds of approximately 70 miles per hour for a short distance.
   cheetah
2. There are two kinds of this animal. The one from Africa is taller and has larger ears than the one from India.
   elephant
3. The young of this mammal are called *joeys* and are the size of a bumblebee when born.
   kangaroo
4. These social animals are the closest relatives to humans, are one of four types of great apes, and can be found in 21 African countries.
   chimpanzee
5. This nocturnal mammal is the only marsupial native to North America. It carries its young in a pouch for about two and half months after birth. Often when danger appears, this animal will fall to its side and appear to be dead.
   opossum
6. This animal, which is not really a bear (although its name includes *bear*), can survive on a diet of eucalyptus leaves.
   koala bear
7. In this family, females are called *sows* and males *boars*. Although we hear otherwise, they would rather stay clean if given the chance.
   pig
8. This animal's height is measured in "hands." One hand equals about 4 inches. Many wear "shoes" on their feet for protection.
   horse
9. This large mammal can spend its whole life on the ice without ever setting foot on land. It feeds on a diet of meat, primarily seals.
   polar bear
10. This animal is the largest animal in existence, lives in the ocean, and is surrounded by a layer of fat called *blubber*. The largest ever recorded was 32 feet long and weighed 22,000 pounds!
    whale
11. This is the only mammal that can fly. They are nocturnal and are not "blind," as some believe they are.
    bat
12. This is the tallest animal in the world, measuring 6 feet when born. It often spreads its legs apart to drink, since its neck is too short to reach the ground otherwise.
    giraffe
13. These animals can spit a distance of 10 feet or more and are members of the camel family. They have been domesticated for thousands of years and are often used as pack animals.
    llama
14. This animal's roar can be heard up to 5 miles away. It lives mostly on the plains of Africa and generally in "prides."
    lion
15. This "sly" animal's most common species is red, although others include gray, arctic, kit and fennec. It is a solitary animal and hunts mostly at night. Its baby is called a *kit*.
    fox
16. This nocturnal animal often invades garbage cans. We often say that they look like "bandits" due to the area around their eyes being a little darker than the rest of their coloring.
    raccoon

FACILITATOR: *Discussions regarding animals could go in so many different directions. How many of these animals have participants seen? Where are some places they could go to see them? What else can they say about them? Pick other animals and ask for interesting facts. Have participants been to a zoo? Do they think it's fair to keep wild animals in captivity? Which animal do they think they are most like? Why?*

Animal Sayings

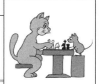

Sayings help us to express our feelings in an unconventional way. Animal sayings are no exception. Perhaps these sayings were created because of the nature of animal behavior, or maybe just because someone was feeling creative. Each of the descriptions below is a clue to a common saying based on a type of animal.

1. A person who eats very little is said to what?

2. When someone lets out a secret, they what?

3. When it rains very heavily, it is said to what?

4. A person who is in trouble is said to be what?

5. When an obvious situation is happening but everyone ignores it, this is said to be a what?

6. When you take care of two things at once, you are said to be able to what?

7. Being able to see things from an aerial point of view is called a what?

8. The hottest days of summer are also called the what?

9. Calling out to someone provocatively is also called a what?

10. It is better to have a small advantage than to risk going for a larger one. This is also called what?

11. If you want someone to slow down, you might tell them to what?

12. To not stir up old conflicts or trouble is to what?

13. When something seems suspicious, you might say that you what?

14. If you don't want someone to get ahead of him- or herself, you would say what?

15. Something that is no good, or that can be dismissed is said to be what?

16. Someone who is stubborn or arrogant is said to be on a what?

17. A very competitive atmosphere or situation is called what?

Animal Sayings ANSWER SHEET

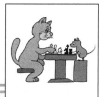

1. A person who eats very little is said to what?
   eat like a bird

2. When someone lets out a secret, they what?
   let the cat out of the bag

3. When it rains very heavily, it is said to what?
   rain cats and dogs

4. A person who is in trouble is said to be what?
   in the doghouse

5. When an obvious situation is happening but everyone ignores it, this is said to be a what?
   elephant in the room

6. When you take care of two things at once, you are said to be able to what?
   kill two birds with one stone

7. Being able to see things from an aerial or overall point of view is called a what?
   bird's eye view

8. The hottest days of summer are also called the what?
   dog days of summer

9. Calling out to someone provocatively is also called a what?
   cat call

10. It is better to have a small advantage than to risk going for a larger one.
    a bird in the hand is worth two in the bush

11. If you want someone to slow down, you might tell him or her to what?
    hold your horses

12. To not stir up old conflicts or trouble is to what?
    let sleeping dogs lie

13. When something seems suspicious, you might say that you what?
    smell a rat

14. If you don't want someone to get ahead of him- or herself, you would say what?
    don't put the cart before the horse

15. Something that is no good, or that can be dismissed is said to be what?
    for the birds

16. Someone who is stubborn or arrogant is said to be on a what?
    high horse

17. A very competitive atmosphere or situation is called what?
    dog eat dog

FACILITATOR: Animals are a fun topic. You can use this worksheet to spur discussion around the following questions: Where do you think these sayings came from? Do the literal translations match the intended meanings? Is it better to use precise English words or phrases instead of sayings, or are there some feelings that come across better when using sayings such as the ones above? What are some others that are not listed above?

The Color of Money

Green is a color we often associate with money in the United States because the paper currency is green. We also associate green with nature, as it is one of the primary colors seen in the great outdoors. The following definitions each describe a word or group of words that contain the word *green*. Can you name each?

1. A note of U.S. currency, especially a dollar.

2. A vegetable similar to scallions.

3. A warm beverage that many drink for medicinal purposes.

4. Someone who is a very good gardener has a what?

5. A place to practice "short" shots in golf.

6. A city in east Wisconsin famous for the Packers.

7. A retail seller of fruits and vegetables.

8. A structure, usually made of glass, in which plants are grown in a temperature-controlled environment.

9. A very large Danish island in the Atlantic Ocean.

10. For drivers, this is a sign that means "okay to proceed."

11. Soldiers from Vermont during the Revolutionary War.

12. Wood before it's altogether seasoned.

13. An expression meaning pale or sickly in appearance.

14. An international environmental group best known for its campaigns against whaling.

15. These vegetables are long and slender and are often called "string."

16. A member of the U.S. Army Special Forces who wears a particular type of hat.

17. A section of parks or an unoccupied area surrounding a community.

18. A card that is issued by the U.S. government to aliens that allows them to work in the United States temporarily.

19. One who has responsibility for keeping up a golf course.

20. An inexperienced person.

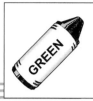

1. A note of U.S. currency, especially a dollar.
   greenback
2. A vegetable similar to scallions.
   green onion
3. A warm beverage that many drink for medicinal purposes.
   green tea
4. Someone who is a very good gardener has a what?
   green thumb
5. A place to practice "short" shots in golf.
   putting green
6. A city in east Wisconsin famous for the Packers.
   Green Bay
7. A retail seller of fruits and vegetables.
   green grocer
8. A structure, usually made of glass, in which plants are grown in a temperature-controlled environment.
   greenhouse
9. A very large Danish island in the Atlantic Ocean.
   Greenland
10. For drivers, this is a sign that means "okay to proceed."
    green light
11. Soldiers from Vermont during the Revolutionary War.
    Green Mountain Boys
12. Wood before it's altogether seasoned.
    green lumber
13. An expression meaning pale or sickly in appearance.
    green around the gills
14. An international environmental group best known for its campaigns against whaling.
    Greenpeace
15. These vegetables are long and slender and are often called "string."
    green beans
16. A member of the U.S. Army Special Forces who wears a particular type of hat.
    Green Beret
17. A section of parks or an unoccupied area surrounding a community.
    greenbelt
18. A card that is issued by the U.S. government to aliens that allows them to work in the United States temporarily.
    green card
19. One who has responsibility for keeping up a golf course.
    greenskeeper
20. An inexperienced person.
    greenhorn

FACILITATOR: *Colors make great conversation starters. Can participants think of any other "green" things? What can they share about these words or expressions? Do they have a green thumb? Do they know anyone who has been a Green Beret? Do they like green tea? Pick another color and ask who can think of words or expressions using that color. If you have time, check out the associations we make with each color. For instance, we often associate sunshine or happiness with yellow.*

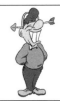

Comedy, Laughter, and Smiles

Laughter is a universal language. It does wonderful things for our bodies and our minds. The following activity deals with laughter and comedy in a variety of ways. How many people, phrases, or words can you identify?

1. These comic performers usually wear colored wigs, outlandish costumes, face paint, and a round red nose.

2. Often heard on television, this soundtrack is made up of the sounds of audience laughter.

3. A laugh that involves much of the body, especially the stomach, is called a what?

4. This comedian traveled the globe during the holidays to entertain U.S. troops for nearly 6 decades.

5. A humorous drawing often with a caption included is called a what?

6. Freddy the Freeloader and Clem Kadiddlehopper were two of this comedian's most famous characters.

7. This comedian was famous for her reporting of American home life in the last half of the 20th century. Her second-favorite household chore was ironing. Her first was hitting her head on the top bunk bed until she fainted.

8. This type of comedy often involves some kind of physical activity, such as that used frequently by The Three Stooges.

9. "My wife Mary and I have been married for 47 years, and not once have we had an argument serious enough to consider divorce. Murder, yes, but divorce, never." This famous quote was made by this comedian about his wife, Mary Livingston.

10. This famous sex symbol was famous for her off-color quotes. She once said, "I generally avoid temptation unless I can't resist it."

11. This cigar-smoking, hard-living star "hated children, dogs, and women, unless they were the wrong sort of women."

12. This is the day of the year when many people trick one another with practical jokes.

13. This is the common name of the elbow and is also an expression defined as one's sense of humor.

14. "One of these days . . . POW, right in the kisser!" was one of this comedian's most famous lines (spoken to his wife, Alice).

15. "Heeeeeere's Johnny!" was the line spoken by Ed McMahon to introduce this man on *The Tonight Show*.

16. "God don't make no mistakes. That's how He got to be God." This is just one of the many famous quotes by this man, who was the star of *All in the Family* in the 1970s.

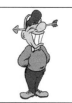

Comedy, Laughter, and Smiles ANSWER SHEET

1. These comic performers usually wear colored wigs, outlandish costumes, face paint, and a round red nose.
    clowns
2. Often heard on television, this soundtrack is made up of the sounds of audience laughter.
    canned laughter (laugh track)
3. A laugh that involves much of the body, especially the stomach, is called a what?
    belly laugh
4. This comedian traveled the globe during the holidays to entertain U.S. troops for nearly 6 decades.
    Bob Hope
5. A humorous drawing often with a caption included is called a what?
    cartoon
6. Freddy the Freeloader and Clem Kadiddlehopper were two of this comedian's most famous characters.
    Red Skelton
7. This comedian was famous for her reporting of American home life in the last half of the 20th century. Her second-favorite household chore was ironing. Her first was hitting her head on the top bunk bed until she fainted.
    Erma Bombeck
8. This type of comedy often involves some kind of physical activity, such as that used frequently by The Three Stooges.
    slapstick
9. "My wife Mary and I have been married for 47 years, and not once have we had an argument serious enough to consider divorce. Murder, yes, but divorce, never." This famous quote was made by this comedian about his wife, Mary Livingston.
    Jack Benny
10. This famous sex symbol was famous for her off-color quotes. She once said, "I generally avoid temptation unless I can't resist it."
    Mae West
11. This cigar-smoking, hard-living star "hated children, dogs, and women, unless they were the wrong sort of women."
    W. C. Fields
12. This is the day of the year when many people trick one another with practical jokes.
    April 1 (April Fools' Day)
13. This is the common name of the elbow and is also an expression defined as one's sense of humor.
    funny bone
14. "One of these days . . . POW, right in the kisser!" was one of this comedian's most famous lines (spoken to his wife, Alice).
    Jackie Gleason
15. "Heeeeeere's Johnny!" was the line spoken by Ed McMahon to introduce this man on *The Tonight Show*.
    Johnny Carson
16. "God don't make no mistakes. That's how He got to be God." This is just one of the many famous quotes by this man, who was the star of *All in the Family* in the 1970s.
    Archie Bunker

FACILITATOR: *This activity should be good for many, many laughs and for wonderful reminiscence. Ask participants to choose their favorite comedian. What is their favorite sitcom? Favorite funny movie? Favorite joke or riddle? Do they consider themselves humorous? What are the benefits of laughter? How important are smiles? You may also want to share some funny stories, pictures, and so forth.*

Events that Changed History

Certain events have the ability to change the course of history, from the early discovery of fire to the Iraq War. These events have occurred over thousands of years in locations throughout the world. Test your knowledge of world history with the following activity, which focuses on some of the events that have changed history in the last few hundred years.

1. This 1989 event, which took place in Germany, signified the end of the Cold War and unified Germany.

2. This war in the late 1700s freed the 13 colonies of the United States from the British Empire.

3. The German invention of this in the 1400s allowed for the widespread availability of the written word.

4. The opening of this waterway in 1914 cut in half the shipping time necessary to go between the Pacific and Atlantic oceans.

5. The 19th Amendment to the U.S. Constitution extended this right to women.

6. The Great Depression of 1929 started with this.

7. Two atomic bombs, the only ones ever to have been detonated, were dropped by the United States on these Japanese cities, killing thousands immediately and more over time.

8. This lunar event during the Cold War in 1969 gave the United States the lead over the Soviet Union in the space race.

9. September 11, 2001, will go down in history for this tragic event, which marked an increased awareness of the threat of terrorism.

10. This man's travels to China in 1298 increased the Western world's awareness that there was a "world" to the east as well.

11. This historic event, which took place in Hawaii in 1941, marked the end of isolationism on the part of the United States.

12. This, the first ten amendments to the U.S. Constitution, limited the power of the federal government and protected the rights of its citizens.

13. This man made the discovery that the Sun, not the Earth, is the center of the universe.

14. U.S., British, and Canadian forces landed on five separate beaches in France in this World War II battle to liberate Europe from Nazi occupation.

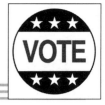

1. This 1989 event, which took place in Germany, signified the end of the Cold War and unified Germany.
    fall of the Berlin Wall

2. This war in the late 1700s freed the 13 colonies of the United States from the British Empire.
    American Revolution

3. The German invention of this in the 1400s allowed for the widespread availability of the written word.
    printing press

4. The opening of this waterway in 1914 cut in half the shipping time necessary to go between the Pacific and Atlantic oceans.
    Panama Canal

5. The 19th Amendment to the U.S. Constitution extended this right to women.
    the right to vote

6. The Great Depression of 1929 started with this.
    Black Monday (stock market crash)

7. Two atomic bombs, the only ones ever to have been detonated, were dropped by the United States on these Japanese cities, killing thousands immediately and more over time.
    Hiroshima and Nagasaki

8. This lunar event during the Cold War in 1969 gave the United States the lead over the Soviet Union in the space race.
    Apollo 11 landing on the Moon

9. September 11, 2001, will go down in history for this tragic event, which marked an increased awareness of the threat of terrorism.
    bombing of the World Trade Center in New York and the Pentagon in Washington, DC

10. This man's travels to China in 1298 increased the Western world's awareness that there was a "world" to the east as well.
    Marco Polo

11. This historic event, which took place in Hawaii in 1941, marked the end of isolationism on the part of the United States.
    bombing of Pearl Harbor

12. This, the first ten amendments to the U.S. Constitution, limited the power of the federal government and protected the rights of its citizens.
    Bill of Rights

13. This man made the discovery that the Sun, not the Earth, is the center of the universe.
    Copernicus

14. U.S., British, and Canadian forces landed on five separate beaches in France in this World War II battle to liberate Europe from Nazi occupation.
    Battle of Normandy (D-Day)

FACILITATOR: *Participants will have lived through many of these events. How many do they remember? Do they remember where they were when they heard about the event? Which other events have changed the course of the world? Which inventions? Which wars? Which discoveries?*

Expressions with Body Parts

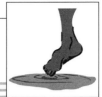

"Get your feet wet" with the following expressions. Below are descriptions of common expressions that include a part of the body. An example is "to jump in and experience something new" (the answer is "get your feet wet"). Keeping in mind body parts, and using the given clues, name as many of these expressions as you can.

1. When a person ignores something that is obviously wrong.
   bury your . . .
2. When something only seems to look good on the surface.
   beauty . . .
3. If a person doesn't react or show any emotion to something.
   doesn't bat . . .
4. If a person shouts something as loudly as he or she can.
   at the . . .
5. When something costs a lot of money.
   an arm . . .
6. When people are constantly arguing and fighting.
   at each . . .
7. Someone who is young and inexperienced.
   wet . . .
8. Someone who is constantly annoying or bothersome.
   pain . . .
9. Someone who is closely following or examining someone else.
   breathing . . .
10. For someone to get his or her first experience at something.
    get your . . .
11. To know a word but not be able to think of it at the moment.
    on the . . .
12. To say something embarrassing or ridiculous.
    put your . . .
13. To start something off incorrectly.
    get off . . .
14. To only imagine something and it's not real.
    all in . . .
15. If everyone is looking at you.
    all eyes . . .
16. When people are apart, their love grows.
    absence . . .
17. Not to have enough space is not to have this.
    elbow . . .
18. To lose the courage to do something.
    get cold . . .
19. To have a strong emotional reaction to something is to be what?
    weak . . .
20. To get rid of a great burden.
    weight . . .

Expressions with Body Parts ANSWER SHEET

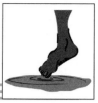

1. When a person ignores something that is obviously wrong.
   bury your head in the sand

2. When something only seems to look good on the surface.
   beauty is only skin deep

3. If a person doesn't react or show any emotion to something.
   doesn't bat an eyelid

4. If a person shouts something as loudly as he or she can.
   at the top of your lungs

5. When something costs a lot of money.
   an arm and a leg

6. When people are constantly arguing and fighting.
   at each others' throats

7. Someone who is young and inexperienced.
   wet behind the ears

8. Someone who is constantly annoying or bothersome.
   pain in the neck

9. Someone who is closely following or examining someone else.
   breathing down your neck

10. For someone to get his or her first experience at something.
    get your feet wet

11. To know a word but not be able to think of it at the moment.
    on the tip of your tongue

12. To say something embarrassing or ridiculous.
    put your foot in your mouth

13. To start something off incorrectly.
    get off on the wrong foot

14. To only imagine something and it's not real.
    all in your head

15. If everyone is looking at you.
    all eyes are on me

16. When people are apart, their love grows.
    absence makes the heart grow fonder

17. Not to have enough space is not to have this.
    elbow room

18. To lose the courage to do something.
    get cold feet

19. To have a strong emotional reaction to something is to be what?
    weak at the knees

20. To get rid of a great burden.
    weight off your shoulders

FACILITATOR: What other expressions do participants know that have body parts? Name a body part such as "thumb" and ask for examples (e.g., "stick out like a sore thumb," "rule of thumb"). How many body parts can they name? Can they make a list from A–Z, naming at least one body part that begins with each letter of the alphabet?

Strengthen Your Mind, Volume Two by Einberger & Sellick. Copyright © 2008 by Health Professions Press, Inc.

Expressions with Colors

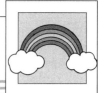

Now that you have the "green light," check out the following expressions, which each include the name of a color. Colors bring vivid pictures to mind and help us to remember information better. For each definition, and using the given color clue, name the expression. For instance, to get the go ahead to do something would be "get the green light" and would have the clue of *green*.

1. When someone talks fast and a great deal.
    blue

2. To go out on the town and have lots of fun.
    red

3. When things look or sound valuable but are not.
    gold

4. When something happens very rarely.
    blue

5. When it's very clear who or what is correct.
    white

6. When you wish very badly that you had what somebody else has.
    green

7. When someone is critical of someone else for something he or she did him- or herself.
    black

8. Sometimes it's better to be silent and not say anything.
    gold

9. To treat someone very special, especially when welcoming him or her.
    red

10. To see things better than what they really are.
    rose

11. To do something over and over again, unsuccessfully.
    blue

12. Do unto others as you would have them do unto you.
    gold

13. To be caught doing something illegal or immoral.
    red

14. To be very pleased with something.
    pink

15. Someone who can make money from anything.
    gold

16. A very loyal and dependable person.
    blue

17. When a person becomes extremely scared.
    white

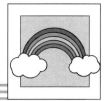

1. When someone talks fast and a great deal.
   talk a blue streak

2. To go out on the town and have lots of fun.
   paint the town red

3. When things look or sound valuable but are not.
   all that glitters is not gold

4. When something happens very rarely.
   once in a blue moon

5. When it's very clear who or what is correct.
   black and white

6. When you wish very badly that you had what somebody else has.
   green with envy

7. When someone is critical of someone else for something he or she did him- or herself.
   the pot calling the kettle black

8. Sometimes it's better to be silent and not say anything.
   silence is golden

9. To treat someone very special, especially when welcoming him or her.
   roll out the red carpet

10. To see things better than what they really are.
    rose-colored glasses

11. To do something over and over again, unsuccessfully.
    till you're blue in the face

12. Do unto others as you would have them do unto you.
    golden rule

13. To be caught doing something illegal or immoral.
    catch someone red-handed

14. To be very pleased with something.
    tickled pink

15. Someone who can make money from anything.
    gold touch

16. A very loyal and dependable person.
    true blue

17. When a person becomes extremely scared.
    white as a sheet

FACILITATOR: *Color can make for a great deal of conversation. Ask participants what comes to mind when they think of a particular color. For instance, does red make them think of anger, or excitement, or pain? Name a particular color and ask participants to identify expressions that go along with that color. For instance, for the color gold there are the expressions "silence is golden" and "a golden handshake."*

Expressions with Foods

The following definitions all offer "food for thought." Each describes a common expression that includes a food item. The name of the food is given as a clue. Can you name the expression?

1. To make oneself look ridiculous or to embarrass oneself.
   egg

2. Someone who earns the money that a family lives on.
   bacon

3. Risking everything on a single opportunity that could go wrong.
   egg

4. Eating this is said to aid in maintaining health.
   apple

5. If someone is caught doing something wrong.
   cookie

6. When someone wants to be involved in something.
   pie

7. A nickname for New York City.
   apple

8. If an idea is utterly impractical.
   pie

9. You shouldn't necessarily believe everything.
   salt

10. If people look or act alike or are always together.
    pea

11. If something is not to one's liking.
    tea

12. If something is selling very quickly.
    cake

13. When someone says something negative or critical.
    grape

14. When it's necessary to tread lightly so as not to anger a person or hurt his or her feelings.
    egg

15. When a person wants everything his or her way, especially if it's contradictory.
    cake

16. If something is very easy to do.
    candy

17. Something one wants, but is immoral or illegal.
    fruit

Expressions with Foods ANSWER SHEET

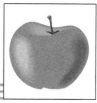

1. To make oneself look ridiculous or to embarrass oneself.
   egg on my face

2. Someone who earns the money that a family lives on.
   bring home the bacon

3. Risking everything on a single opportunity that could go wrong.
   put all your eggs in one basket

4. Eating this is said to aid in maintaining health.
   an apple a day keeps the doctor away

5. If someone is caught doing something wrong.
   caught with your hands in the cookie jar

6. When someone wants to be involved in something.
   finger in the pie

7. A nickname for New York City.
   Big Apple

8. If an idea is utterly impractical.
   pie in the sky

9. You shouldn't necessarily believe everything.
   grain of salt

10. If people look or act alike or are always together.
    peas in a pod

11. If something is not to one's liking.
    not your cup of tea

12. If something is selling very quickly.
    like hot cakes

13. When someone says something negative or critical.
    sour grapes

14. When it's necessary to tread lightly so as not to anger a person or hurt his or her feelings.
    walk on eggshells

15. When a person wants everything his or her way, especially if it's contradictory.
    can't have your cake and eat it, too

16. If something is very easy to do.
    taking candy from a baby

17. Something one wants, but is immoral or illegal.
    forbidden fruit

FACILITATOR: *Food often brings taste and smell to mind. Discuss this fact with participants. What tastes and smells do these sayings bring to mind? Do they really make sense? Can anyone guess how the expressions might have been started? Do they know of any other expressions that use foods?*

Strengthen Your Mind, Volume Two by Einberger & Sellick. Copyright © 2008 by Health Professions Press, Inc.

Expressions with Numbers

Go "the whole nine yards" in figuring out the common expressions described below. Each has a number expressed in a certain way—as a whole number, as money, as a measurement. For example, when someone does something completely, he or he has gone "the whole nine yards." A clue is given with each definition.

1. To give an opinion on an issue.
   two

2. To first try to understand someone before criticizing him or her.
   mile

3. If people look or act alike or are always together.
   two

4. Something that is very, very common and, at times, too common.
   dozen

5. Someone who is careful with small amounts of money but careless with larger amounts.
   pound

6. When a person has consumed a great deal of alcohol.
   three

7. When a person is willing to go above and beyond for someone else.
   mile

8. When something is too little, too late.
   dollar

9. To advise someone not to allow him- or herself to be taken advantage of.
   nickels

10. To put things off until the last minute.
    eleventh

11. Someone or something unnecessary or useless.
    fifth

12. When something specific happens a lot.
    nickel

13. When all members of a group pledge to support each of the individual members, and the individual members pledge to support the group.
    one

14. When two options are similar and neither is better than the other.
    six

15. It's better to do something right the first time so that it won't cost more time later.
    nine

16. To risk everything instead of spreading the risk.
    one

17. To put someone under a great deal of pressure to tell the truth about something.
    third

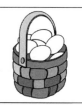

1. To give an opinion on an issue.
   two cents worth

2. To first try to understand someone before criticizing him or her.
   walk a mile in his or her shoes

3. If people look or act alike or are always together.
   two peas in a pod

4. Something that is very, very common and, at times, too common.
   dime a dozen

5. Someone who is careful with small amounts of money but careless with larger amounts.
   penny-wise, pound-foolish

6. When a person has consumed a great deal of alcohol.
   three sheets to the wind

7. When a person is willing to go above and beyond for someone else.
   go the extra mile

8. When something is too little, too late.
   a day late and a dollar short

9. To advise someone not to allow him- or herself to be taken advantage of.
   don't take any wooden nickels

10. To put things off until the last minute.
    eleventh hour

11. Someone or something unnecessary or useless.
    fifth wheel

12. When something specific happens a lot.
    if I had a nickel for every time . . .

13. When all members of a group pledge to support each of the individual members, and the individual members pledge to support the group.
    all for one and one for all

14. When two options are similar and neither is better than the other.
    six of one and a half dozen of another

15. It's better to do something right the first time so that it won't cost more time later.
    a stitch in time saves nine

16. To risk everything instead of spreading the risk.
    put all your eggs in one basket

17. To put someone under a great deal of pressure to tell the truth about something.
    third degree

FACILITATOR: *Ask participants which of these expressions they use the most. What does each expression mean to them? Are there other expressions that they use frequently? How do they think the numbers in each expression came to be used?*

Fabulous in Fives

We are surrounded in everyday life by things that come in fives—increments of money, days of the workweek, fingers on our hands, and toes on our feet. Get your fill of fives by trying this worksheet. Most of the answers will have the word *five* in them.

1. Another name for a variety store, this type of retailer sells items for a very low cost.

2. On the Saffir-Simpson Hurricane Scale, the most powerful hurricanes are given this rating.

3. In musical notation, the staff symbol is made of four spaces and what?

4. This symbol of the Olympic Games is made up of five loops, each a different color.

5. In the sport of hockey, if a player shoots a puck between the legs of the goaltender, it is called a what?

6. On a standard telephone, what letters of the alphabet are listed on the keypad number 5?

7. Sweet, sour, bitter, salty, and umami are commonly known as what?

8. Which president is pictured on the five-dollar bill?

9. Five children born at once are called what?

10. In music, this is considered one of the most important intervals other than the octave.

11. In this sport, only five players are allowed on the court at a time.

12. In radio communication, this expression is similar to "loud and clear."

13. Another name for a car with a manual transmission is a what?

14. These fragrant flowers are known for having five petals.

15. It is commonly known that humans have five senses. Can you list them?

16. The world has five oceans. Can you list them?

17. Air, earth, fire, water, and wood are known as the what?

18. In biology, all living things are divided into one of the what?

19. A pentagram is also called a what?

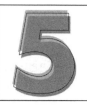

1. Another name for a variety store, this type of retailer sells items for a very low cost.
    five-and-dime

2. On the Saffir-Simpson Hurricane Scale, the most powerful hurricanes are given this rating.
    category 5

3. In musical notation, the staff symbol is made of four spaces and what?
    five horizontal lines

4. This symbol of the Olympic Games is made up of five loops, each a different color.
    Olympic Rings

5. In the sport of hockey, if a player shoots a puck between the legs of the goaltender, it is called a what?
    five-hole

6. On a standard telephone, what letters of the alphabet are listed on the keypad number 5?
    J, K, L

7. Sweet, sour, bitter, salty, and umami are commonly known as what?
    five tastes

8. Which president is pictured on the five-dollar bill?
    Abraham Lincoln

9. Five children born at once are called what?
    quintuplets

10. In music, this is considered one of the most important intervals other than the octave.
    perfect fifth

11. In this sport, only five players are allowed on the court at a time.
    basketball

12. In radio communication, this expression is similar to "loud and clear."
    five by five

13. Another name for a car with a manual transmission is a what?
    five-speed

14. These fragrant flowers are known for having five petals.
    roses

15. It is commonly known that humans have five senses. Can you list them?
    hearing, sight, smell, taste, touch

16. The world has five oceans. Can you list them?
    Pacific, Atlantic, Indian, Artic, Antarctic

17. Air, earth, fire, water, and wood are known as the what?
    five elements

18. In biology, all living things are divided into one of the what?
    five kingdoms

19. A pentagram is also called a what?
    five-pointed star

FACILITATOR: *Working with numbers is a fun and mentally challenging activity, especially for math buffs! Ask participants to list as many things that come in fives as they can (there are many more that are not on the worksheet). For extra mental exercise, ask the group to think of some mathematical equations that equal the number five. What number is five the root of? Is five anyone's lucky number? If not, what is everyone's lucky number?*

Famous Brand-Names

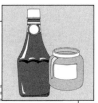

There are thousands of brand-names in the food industry. Many companies make a variety of foods. Some make only one. The following companies are especially well known for producing one certain product. Can you name that product?

1. Gold Medal

2. Campbell's

3. C&H

4. Arm & Hammer

5. Duncan Hines

6. Sara Lee

7. Smucker's

8. Lipton

9. Oscar Meyer

10. Jimmy Dean

11. Chicken of the Sea

12. Ocean Spray

13. Quaker

14. Uncle Ben's

15. Lee & Perrins

16. Dole

17. Tillamook

18. Log Cabin

19. Heinz

20. Best Foods

21. Ragu

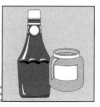

1. Gold Medal
    flour
2. Campbell's
    soup
3. C&H
    sugar
4. Arm & Hammer
    baking soda
5. Duncan Hines
    cake and brownie mixes
6. Sara Lee
    desserts
7. Smucker's
    jams and jellies
8. Lipton
    tea
9. Oscar Meyer
    hot dogs
10. Jimmy Dean
    sausage
11. Chicken of the Sea
    tuna
12. Ocean Spray
    cranberry and other juices
13. Quaker
    oatmeal
14. Uncle Ben's
    rice
15. Lea & Perrins
    Worcestershire sauce
16. Dole
    pineapple and other fruits
17. Tillamook
    cheese
18. Log Cabin
    syrup
19. Heinz
    ketchup
20. Best Foods
    mayonnaise
21. Ragu
    spaghetti sauce

FACILITATOR: *There are many, many other food brands that are especially known for one product. How many can participants name? Which have they tried? Do they think brand-names are always better? Do they think it's worth the extra cost to purchase brand-names? Why do brand-names cost more? It would be fun actually to have some well-known brand-name products on hand. You might want to have a couple of taste tests—store-brand cereal versus brand-name, or store-brand ice-cream versus brand-name.*

Famous Recipes

Some recipes are so delicious that they become an instant, timeless favorite. Many of us grew up eating these recipes, most of which were printed on the back of food boxes or bags. Wet your palate by reading the descriptions below—and have a snack on hand in case you get hungry!

1. This famous treat requires only three ingredients: crisp cereal, marshmallows, and butter.

2. Famous during the Fall season, this pumpkin pie recipe is printed on the back of this brand of canned pumpkin.

3. This salty snack mix is made from corn, rice, and wheat cereal and can include pretzels, peanuts, and several seasonings.

4. Adding two cups of sour cream to this famous dip mix makes for a delicious snack treat.

5. Campbell's makes the most famous version of this "feel better" recipe, but many a grandmother has had her own recipe as well.

6. Making biscuits using this mix is a breeze using the recipe printed on the back of the box.

7. Originally coined "America's Most Favorite Dessert," this wiggly treat can be molded into many forms.

8. Traditionally eaten around the holidays, this rich recipe calls for dried and/or candied fruit, spices, and nuts and is often soaked in brandy.

9. Invented in 1930 at a restaurant in Massachusetts, you can still find the recipe for these cookies on the back of the bag of chocolate chips.

10. In 1955, this recipe was first printed on the back of a can of Campbell's cream of mushroom soup. Today, many people enjoy this vegetable casserole around the holidays.

11. Sometimes called a brown cow, this cool treat has many variations but is traditionally made of root beer and ice-cream.

12. English people often eat this bread-like food, made of flour and egg, with roast beef.

13. This delicious cake is traditionally made with chocolate and has coconut sprinkled over the top and sides.

14. This popular breakfast food consists of an English muffin, bacon or ham, eggs, and hollandaise sauce.

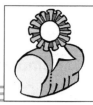

1. This famous treat requires only three ingredients: crisp cereal, marshmallows, and butter.
   Rice Krispies Treats

2. Famous during the Fall season, this pumpkin pie recipe is printed on the back of this brand of canned pumpkin.
   Libby's

3. This salty snack mix is made from corn, rice, and wheat cereal and can include pretzels, peanuts, and several seasonings.
   Chex Mix

4. Adding two cups of sour cream to this famous dip mix makes for a delicious snack treat.
   Lipton onion dip

5. Campbell's makes the most famous version of this "feel better" recipe, but many a grandmother has had her own recipe as well.
   chicken soup

6. Making biscuits using this mix is a breeze using the recipe printed on the back of the box.
   Bisquick

7. Originally coined "America's Most Favorite Dessert," this wiggly treat can be molded into many forms.
   jello

8. Traditionally eaten around the holidays, this rich recipe calls for dried and/or candied fruit, spices, and nuts and is often soaked in brandy.
   fruitcake

9. Invented in 1930 at a restaurant in Massachusetts, you can still find the recipe for these cookies on the back of the bag of chocolate chips.
   Nestlé Toll House chocolate chip cookies

10. In 1955, this recipe was first printed on the back of a can of Campbell's cream of mushroom soup. Today, many people enjoy this vegetable casserole around the holidays.
    green bean casserole

11. Sometimes called a brown cow, this cool treat has many variations but is traditionally made of root beer and ice-cream.
    root beer float

12. English people often eat this bread-like food, made of flour and egg, with roast beef.
    Yorkshire pudding

13. This delicious cake is traditionally made with chocolate and has coconut sprinkled over the top and sides.
    German chocolate cake

14. This popular breakfast food consists of an English muffin, bacon or ham, eggs, and hollandaise sauce.
    eggs Benedict

FACILITATOR: *Enjoyment of foods can bring back many memories. How many of you have eaten these foods? Are there certain seasons or holidays during which these recipes were enjoyed? What are some attributes that these foods have that make them famous? What recipes in your family are considered "famous"?*

Food around the United States

People in different countries around the world eat food particular to their culture. Italians eat a lot of pasta. People in Mexico often eat beans, tortillas, and cheese. The Chinese eat a great deal of rice. People in the United States also have some common tastes for foods. Different areas of the country are known for a particular food or drink. Can you name the state or city known for the following regional specialties?

1. baked beans   _____
2. lobster   _____
3. oranges   _____
4. cheese   _____
5. apples   _____
6. coconut   _____
7. Cajun   _____
8. sourdough French bread   _____
9. world-class wine   _____
10. clam chowder   _____
11. bourbon   _____
12. Ghirardelli chocolate   _____
13. King salmon   _____
14. potatoes   _____
15. poi   _____
16. Coors beer   _____
17. Café du Mond beignets   _____
18. maple syrup   _____
19. barbeque   _____
20. cheese steak   _____
21. Coney Island hot dog   _____
22. bagels   _____
23. deep-dish pizza   _____
24. gumbo   _____
25. coffee milk   _____
26. buffalo wings   _____
27. key lime pie   _____
28. Derby Pie   _____
29. spiedies   _____
30. shoofly pie   _____
31. johnnycake   _____
32. California roll   _____
33. po' boy sandwich   _____
34. hot brown   _____
35. jambalaya   _____
36. grits   _____
37. crab cakes   _____
38. kalua pig   _____

Food around the United States ANSWER SHEET

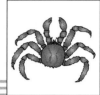

1.	baked beans	**Boston**
2.	lobster	**Maine**
3.	oranges	**Florida**
4.	cheese	**Wisconsin and California**
5.	apples	**Washington**
6.	coconut	**Hawaii**
7.	Cajun	**New Orleans**
8.	sourdough French bread	**San Francisco**
9.	world-class wine	**Napa Valley**
10.	clam chowder	**Boston**
11.	bourbon	**Kentucky**
12.	Ghirardelli chocolate	**San Francisco**
13.	King salmon	**Alaska**
14.	potatoes	**Idaho**
15.	poi	**Hawaii**
16.	Coors beer	**Golden, Colorado**
17.	Café du Mond beignets	**New Orleans**
18.	maple syrup	**Vermont**
19.	barbeque	**Texas and Kansas City**
20.	cheese steak	**Philadelphia**
21.	Coney Island hot dog	**New York**
22.	bagels	**New York**
23.	deep-dish pizza	**Chicago**
24.	gumbo	**Louisiana**
25.	coffee milk	**Rhode Island**
26.	buffalo wings	**New York**
27.	key lime pie	**Florida**
28.	Derby Pie	**Kentucky**
29.	spiedies	**New York**
30.	shoofly pie	**Pennsylvania**
31.	johnnycake	**Rhode Island**
32.	California roll	**Los Angeles**
33.	po' boy sandwich	**Louisiana**
34.	hot brown	**Kentucky**
35.	jambalaya	**Louisiana**
36.	grits	**South Carolina**
37.	crab cakes	**Maryland**
38.	kalua pig	**Hawaii**

FACILITATOR: *You might want to have a couple of these foods available for added fun. Which of these do the participants like best? What do they think made these areas famous for these foods? Are there certain foods or drinks that each participant's state or city is known for? Can they think of other regional foods or drinks? Is there a particular brand associated with any of them?*

Strengthen Your Mind, Volume Two by Einberger & Sellick. Copyright © 2008 by Health Professions Press, Inc.

Important Dates in History

Certain dates have gone down in history as being very important worldwide. Some dates have a very large impact on each of us personally. Can you name the event that made these dates memorable? A location is given as a clue for some dates.

1. July 20, 1969 (far, far away!)

2. 1959 (western United States)

3. December 7, 1941

4. July 4, 1776

5. September 11, 2001

6. 1963 (Dallas)

7. October 12, 1492 (eastern United States)

8. November 1989 (Germany)

9. April 12, 1861 (Ft. Sumter)

10. June 6, 1944 (France)

11. 1939

12. October 29, 1929 (New York)

13. August 26, 1920 (Kitty Hawk, North Carolina)

14. 1914

15. December 17, 1903 (U.S. Congress)

16. 1607 (Virginia)

17. 1954 (U.S. Supreme Court)

18. 1968 (Memphis and Los Angeles)

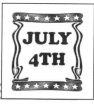

1. July 20, 1969 (far, far away!)
    Neil Armstrong became the first human to walk on the Moon.

2. 1959 (western United States)
    Alaska and Hawaii became the 49th and 50th states.

3. December 7, 1941
    Pearl Harbor, Hawaii, was attacked by Japan.

4. July 4, 1776
    The Continental Congress met in Philadelphia to sign the Declaration of Independence.

5. September 11, 2001
    Terrorists crashed hijacked planes into the New York World Trade Center and the Pentagon.

6. 1963 (Dallas)
    John F. Kennedy was assassinated in Houston, Texas.

7. October 12, 1492 (eastern United States)
    Christopher Columbus landed in the New World after setting sail from Spain with the Niña, the Pinta, and the Santa Maria.

8. November 1989 (Germany)
    The Berlin Wall between East and West Germany fell.

9. April 12, 1861 (Ft. Sumter)
    The Confederacy attacked the U.S. Army Post at Ft. Sumter, beginning the Civil War.

10. June 6, 1944 (France)
    General Eisenhower led the Allied invasion of Normandy on this day, D-Day.

11. 1939
    Germany invaded Poland, beginning World War II.

12. October 29, 1929 (New York)
    The New York Stock Market crashed on this day, Black Tuesday.

13. August 26, 1920 (U.S. Congress)
    The 19th amendment was signed, giving women the right to vote.

14. 1914
    Archduke Franz Ferdinand of Austria–Hungary was assassinated, beginning World War I.

15. December 17, 1903 (Kitty Hawk, North Carolina)
    The Wright Brothers made the first flight, remaining in the air for 12 seconds.

16. 1607 (Virginia)
    The English began their first settlement in the United States in Jamestown, Virginia.

17. 1954 (U.S. Supreme Court)
    The Supreme Court ordered an end to school segregation.

18. 1968 (Memphis and Los Angeles)
    Martin Luther King Jr. was assassinated in Memphis, Tennessee and Robert F. Kennedy was assassinated in Los Angeles, California.

FACILITATOR: *These are just a few of the most important dates in history. Which others can participants name? On which of these dates do they remember where they were? What impact did these events have on local, U.S., and world history? You might want to have participants make a time line of important dates in their lifetimes.*

In the Dark

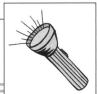

Get out your flashlights, it's dark outside! While most of our waking hours are spent in the light, there are many situations that call for the absence of light. Whether you are afraid of the dark or not, this worksheet explores all things dim in color.

1. When the Moon is invisible from Earth and the night sky is at its darkest.

2. A formal party with formal dress.

3. Another name for when the power goes out.

4. This city in Virginia is the home of the Virginia Polytechnic Institute, or Virginia Tech.

5. This game is played in the night darkness and is a variation of traditional tag.

6. A room specifically designed for developing photographs.

7. Many outdoor recreational settings have this type of surface for playing games and sports.

8. In Europe, the period of time after the fall of the Roman Empire when there was little prosperity is called this.

9. In car racing, this is used to signal the racers to return to their pit area.

10. A person who likes to stay up late and be active at night.

11. During Winter certain cities in this state are in darkness for up to 24 hours.

12. A company that is free of debt is said to be in the what?

13. In politics, a little-known candidate who is expected to win is a what?

14. When a person is unaware or unknowing, he or she is said to be what?

15. A person who is afraid of the dark might have one of these lights in his or her room.

In the Dark ANSWER SHEET

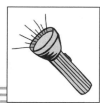

1. When the Moon is invisible from Earth and the night sky is at its darkest.
   new Moon

2. A formal party with formal dress.
   black-tie

3. Another name for when the power goes out.
   blackout

4. This city in Virginia is the home of the Virginia Polytechnic Institute, or Virginia Tech.
   Blacksburg

5. This game is played in the night darkness and is a variation of traditional tag.
   flashlight tag

6. A room specifically designed for developing photographs.
   darkroom

7. Many outdoor recreational settings have this type of surface for playing games and sports.
   blacktop

8. In Europe, the period of time after the fall of the Roman Empire when there was little prosperity is called this.
   Dark Ages

9. In car racing, this is used to signal the racers to return to their pit area.
   black flag

10. A person who likes to stay up late and be active at night.
    night owl

11. During Winter certain cities in this state are in darkness for up to 24 hours.
    Alaska

12. A company that is free of debt is said to be what?
    in the black

13. In politics, a little-known candidate who is expected to win is a what?
    dark horse

14. When a person is unaware or unknowing, he or she is said to be what?
    in the dark

15. A person who is afraid of the dark might have one of these lights in his or her room.
    night-light

FACILITATOR: *This worksheet will bring up discussion about the color black. What is the definition of black? What does the color black signify? What do participants think about young people who dress in all black? What about other colors—blue, green, or yellow? Have any participants ever been afraid of the dark? What did they do about it?*

In the Middle of Things

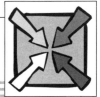

The words *middle* and *mid* are used in a variety of ways. We often speak of being "in the middle of something," of being a "middle child," of losing a thought in "mid-sentence," and so forth. The following definitions all refer to words or phrases that have either the word "middle" or "mid" in them. Can you name each?

1. When parents don't get along, children are often what?

2. Pursuing a course of action that is midway between extremes is called taking the what?

3. Some people go through a difficult time during their 40s. They are said to be having a what?

4. A popular comedy by Shakespeare is what?

5. A big exam in the middle of a school semester is called a what?

6. An often-heard expression advising against change is "Don't change horses in" what?

7. Six is half way between 0 and 12. Therefore, it is the what?

8. Another word for 12:00 a.m. is what?

9. A woman who assists in childbirth is called a what?

10. People who are neither poor nor rich but somewhere in between are often said to be in the what?

11. Southwest Asia and Northeast Africa are considered the what?

12. A point of view between two different opinions is called the what?

13. Another name for junior high school is what?

14. A person who acts as the intermediary between the producer and the consumer is called a what?

15. If we're sharing a piece of pie equally, we need to cut it where?

16. If we travel far out of our way and are not near anything familiar, we are where?

17. If something is above ground level, it is said to be where?

18. The period of history before the Renaissance is called the what?

19. The area of a fair or circus where the sideshows are held is called the what?

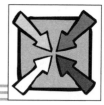

1. When parents don't get along, children are often what?
    caught in the middle

2. Pursuing a course of action that is midway between extremes is called taking the what?
    middle of the road

3. Some people go through a difficult time during their 40s. They are said to be having a what?
    midlife crisis

4. A popular comedy by Shakespeare is what?
    A Midsummer Night's Dream

5. A big exam in the middle of a school semester is called a what?
    midterm

6. An often-heard expression advising against change is "Don't change horses in" what?
    midstream

7. Six is half way between 0 and 12. Therefore, it is the what?
    midpoint

8. Another word for 12:00 a.m. is what?
    midnight

9. A woman who assists in childbirth is called a what?
    midwife

10. People who are neither poor nor rich but somewhere in between are often said to be in the what?
    middle class

11. Southwest Asia and Northeast Africa are considered the what?
    Middle East

12. A point of view between two different opinions is called the what?
    middle ground

13. Another name for junior high school is what?
    middle school

14. A person who acts as the intermediary between the producer and the consumer is called a what?
    middle man

15. If we're sharing a piece of pie equally, we need to cut it where?
    down the middle

16. If we travel far out of our way and are not near anything familiar, we are where?
    middle of nowhere

17. If something is above ground level, it is said to be where?
    midair

18. The period of history before the Renaissance is called the what?
    Middle Ages

19. The area of a fair or circus where the sideshows are held is called the what?
    midway

FACILITATOR: *Discuss each answer as appropriate for further explanation and clarification. Which other words or phrases can participants think of that have the words middle or mid in them? How does it feel to be the middle child, in the middle of an argument, in a midlife crisis? Has anyone ever been caught in the middle of anything?*

Man's Best Friend

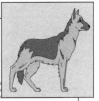

Dogs are commonly referred to as "man's best friend." Indeed, for many of us they make wonderful pets. This activity relates to dogs in a variety of ways. Some questions ask for more than one answer, some for expressions that contain the word *dog*, and others simply ask for facts. How many questions can you answer?

1. This dog has been the most commonly registered dog in the United States since 1991.

2. Besides being used as wonderful pets, name four other uses for dogs.

3. Name three famous dogs, either real or fictional.

4. What is the name of Dorothy's dog in *The Wizard of Oz*?

5. A person who is in charge of an entire operation is often called the what?

6. This is the name of a popular book written by Jack London about a wild dog's journey in Canada.

7. A popular song of the early 1950s, Patti Page sung of wanting to know the cost of a dog.

8. This is an annual sled dog race held in Alaska that takes at least 8 days to complete.

9. This book, written by John Steinbeck, documents a road trip he took with his dog.

10. What are the most popular names for dogs in the United States?

11. When a person is very ill, we often say that he or she is what?

12. Dogs are in this family of animals.

13. Name two breeds of dog that are very large.

14. Name two breeds of dog that are very small.

15. What is the world's fastest dog?

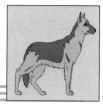

1. This dog has been the most commonly registered dog in the United States since 1991.
   Labrador Retriever

2. Besides being used as wonderful pets, name four other uses for dogs.
   guide dog, police dog, rescue dog, guard dog, therapy dog, hunting dog, herding dog

3. Name three famous dogs, either real or fictional
   Rin Tin Tin, Lassie, Eddie, Fido, Benji, Buddy (President Bill Clinton's dog), Snoopy, Old Yeller

4. What is the name of Dorothy's dog in *The Wizard of Oz*?
   Toto

5. A person who is in charge of an entire operation is often called the what?
   top dog

6. This is the name of a popular book written by Jack London about a wild dog's journey in Canada
   White Fang

7. A popular song of the early 1950s, Patti Page sung of wanting to know the cost of a dog.
   "How Much Is that Doggie in the Window?"

8. This is an annual sled dog race held in Alaska that takes at least 8 days to complete.
   Iditarod Trail Sled Dog Race

9. This book, written by John Steinbeck, documents a road trip he took with his dog.
   Travels with Charley

10. What are the most popular names for dogs in the United States?
    In 2004 Veterinary Pet Insurance listed Max, Jake, Bailey, Cody, and Bear as the top 5 male names for dogs and Molly, Daisy, Sadie, Chloe, and Sophie as the top 5 female names. Other top names include Sam, Lady, Maggie, Buddy, Tasha, Chelsea, Holly, and Shasta.

11. When a person is very ill, we often say that he or she is what?
    sick as a dog

12. Dogs are in this family of animals.
    canine

13. Name two breeds of dog that are very large.
    Newfoundland, Old English Mastiff, Irish Wolfhound, Great Dane, St. Bernard, Great Pyrenees, and so forth

14. Name two breeds of dog that are very small.
    Chihuahua, Pekingese, Toy Fox Terrier, Dachshund, Papillon, Pomeranian, Shih Tzu, Yorkshire Terrier, and so forth

15. What is the world's fastest dog?
    Greyhound

FACILITATOR: *This is a good activity for participants to talk about their pets, both current ones and ones they had in the past. How many think dogs are the best pets? What other facts regarding dogs do they know? Which breed of dog do they think is the best pet, the best guard dog, or the best protector?*

Mothers and Fathers

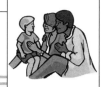

We often use the terms *mother* and *father* for someone or something other than our male or female parent. Below you will find definitions of commonly used names and phrases that pertain to nature, history, religion, and so forth. Each name or phrase has the word *mother* or *father*. Can you name each?

1.   A word often used for a mother who can do everything—take care of the home, take the children to soccer, have a full-time job, and more.

2.   An often-used phrase to describe the creation of something new ("Necessity is the . . . ").

3.   Santa Claus in England is called what?

4.   Wildlife, weather, flora, and fauna are often referred to as what?

5.   This male figure is usually seen carrying an hourglass.

6.   A woman who bears a child for a woman who is unable to do so is called a what?

7.   This woman (or some would say bird!) wrote nursery rhymes.

8.   George Washington was known as this.

9.   One's native land is called what?

10.   The Virgin Mother is sometimes called what?

11.   The leading figures in the founding of the United States are called what?

12.   The nun in charge of a religious order is called this.

13.   A man, often older, who embodies the ideal male parent is often called a what?

14.   Another name for one's native language is what?

15.   This Roman Catholic nun from India won a Nobel Peace Prize for her humanitarian work.

16.   This painting now hangs in an art museum in Paris and is a portrait of the artist's mother.

17.   A female leader of a Cub Scout troop is called a what?

18.   This woman, made famous in a nursery rhyme, went to the cupboard to find her poor dog a bone.

19.   This game, often played in childhood, requests permission to "take two steps."

20.   This is an area where silver or gold is mined. The Sierra Foothills in California, where gold was discovered, is especially known as this.

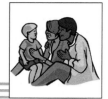

1. A word often used for a mother who can do everything—take care of the home, take the children to soccer, have a full-time job, and more.
   supermom
2. An often-used phrase to describe the creation of something new ("Necessity is the . . . ").
   mother of invention
3. Santa Claus in England is called what?
   Father Christmas
4. Wildlife, weather, flora, and fauna are often referred to as what?
   Mother Nature
5. This male figure is usually seen carrying an hourglass.
   Father Time
6. A woman who bears a child for a woman who is unable to do so is called a what?
   surrogate mother
7. This woman (or some would say bird!) wrote nursery rhymes.
   Mother Goose
8. George Washington was known as this.
   Father of the Country
9. One's native land is called what?
   motherland
10. The Virgin Mother is sometimes called what?
    Mother of God or Mother Mary
11. The leading figures in the founding of the United States are called what?
    Founding Fathers
12. The nun in charge of a religious order is called this.
    Mother Superior
13. A man, often older, who embodies the ideal male parent is often called a what?
    father figure
14. Another name for one's native language is what?
    mother tongue
15. This Roman Catholic nun from India won a Nobel Peace Prize for her humanitarian work.
    Mother Teresa
16. This painting now hangs in an art museum in Paris and is a portrait of the artist's mother.
    Whistler's Mother
17. A female leader of a Cub Scout troop is called a what?
    den mother
18. This woman, made famous in a nursery rhyme, went to the cupboard to find her poor dog a bone.
    Old Mother Hubbard
19. This game, often played in childhood, requests permission to "take two steps."
    Mother, May I?
20. This is an area where silver or gold is mined. The Sierra Foothills in California, where gold was discovered, is especially known as this.
    mother lode

FACILITATOR: *This activity provides a perfect opportunity for participants to talk about their parents and to discuss special memories. Talk about each answer. What else can participants tell you about the father of our country, the mother lode, Whistler's Mother, and so forth? Were any of the female participants ever a den mother or a super-mom? Were any of the male participants a father figure to anyone or did they themselves have a father figure?*

Over and Under

We use the words *over* and *under* to denote position (something that is above or below something else). We also use *over* and *under* to describe emotions, with expressions, and in a variety of other ways. The following definitions are for words or phrases that contain either the word *over* or *under*. How many can you name?

1. The method by which a pitcher throws the ball in slow-pitch softball.

2. Legend has it that a pot of gold is located here.

3. Where gophers live.

4. When something is said to be better than it really is.

5. To do something that is secret or not straightforward.

6. A person who is not old enough to drink legally.

7. When a person takes more than the prescribed amount of a medication.

8. When a person responds in a manner that is unnecessary or with inappropriate emotion.

9. A person who does not eat enough to be healthy.

10. When a person "goes the extra mile."

11. Someone who is domineering.

12. A college student who has not yet received a bachelor's degree.

13. When there is too much light in a photograph.

14. When a person writes a check without having enough money in his or her account.

15. One who is expected to lose a contest or sporting event, but who may actually win.

16. When someone is engaged in spying or a secret investigation.

17. When a yard has many weeds and has not been trimmed in some time.

18. An unintentional omission.

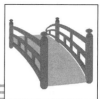

1. The method by which a pitcher throws the ball in slow-pitch softball.
    underhand

2. Legend has it that a pot of gold is located here.
    over the rainbow

3. Where gophers live.
    underground

4. When something is said to be better than it really is.
    overrated

5. To do something that is secret or not straightforward.
    under the table

6. A person who is not old enough to drink legally.
    underage

7. When a person takes more than the prescribed amount of a medication.
    overdose

8. When a person responds in a manner that is unnecessary or with inappropriate emotion.
    overreact

9. A person who does not eat enough to be healthy.
    undernourished

10. When a person "goes the extra mile."
    over and above

11. Someone who is domineering.
    overbearing

12. A college student who has not yet received a bachelor's degree.
    undergraduate

13. When there is too much light in a photograph.
    overexposed

14. When a person writes a check without having enough money in his or her account.
    overdraw

15. One who is expected to lose a contest or sporting event, but who may actually win.
    underdog

16. When someone is engaged in spying or a secret investigation.
    undercover

17. When a yard has many weeds and has not been trimmed in some time.
    overgrown

18. An unintentional omission.
    oversight

FACILITATOR: *Words and phrases that have over and under are plentiful. These are just a few. How many more can participants name? Discuss some of the words and ask for their comments. Do they ever overreact to situations? Have they ever been overdrawn at the bank? Can they think of a time when they have gone over and above? What was the result? How many phrases, such as under/overbid or over/underdress, can they name in which either under or over could be used, giving the phrase opposite meanings?*

Pass the Cheese, Please!

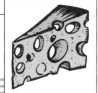

Charles de Gaulle once asked, "How can you govern a country in which there are 246 kinds of cheese?" There are actually hundreds more than this in different parts of the world. Answers to the following questions include some type of cheese as well as facts related to cheese. Test your cheese knowledge with this activity!

1. A type of cheese known for its very powerful smell.

2. This cheese was first made in England and is the most popular cheese in that country. It usually comes in a variety of forms, including mild, medium, and sharp.

3. Which two states are the biggest producers of cheese?

4. What is the expression often used when people are having their picture taken and the photographer wants them to smile?

5. Which country is the world's largest producer of cheese?

6. What are some common foods consumed in the United States that contain cheese?

7. A coarse, lightweight cotton fabric sometimes used to wrap cheese.

8. Name two animals from whose milk cheese is made.

9. An American slang word that means "of poor quality."

10. Which country consumes the most cheese?

11. This dish, which originated in Switzerland, is made from melted cheese into which bread is dipped.

12. This pale yellow cheese contains many holes.

13. This hard, dry Italian cheese is usually grated over pasta dishes.

14. People often eat cheese in order to get a sufficient amount of this in their diet. It is especially good for strong bones.

15. This mild, very soft cheese, made from curds, is often served with pineapple.

16. Wisconsin's Green Bay Packers fans are often called this!

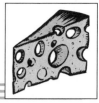

1. A type of cheese known for its very powerful smell.
   Limburger

2. This cheese was first made in England and is the most popular cheese in that country. It usually comes in a variety of forms, including mild, medium, and sharp.
   cheddar

3. Which two states are the biggest producers of cheese?
   California and Wisconsin

4. What is the expression often used when people are having their picture taken and the photographer wants them to smile?
   say cheese!

5. Which country is the world's largest producer of cheese?
   United States (30% of the total), followed by Germany and France

6. What are some common foods consumed in the United States that contain cheese?
   sandwiches, macaroni and cheese, pizza, omelets, lasagna, cheesecake

7. A coarse, lightweight cotton fabric sometimes used to wrap cheese.
   cheesecloth

8. Name at least two animals from whose milk cheese is made.
   cows, sheep, goats, buffalo, and other mammals

9. An American slang word that means "of poor quality."
   cheesy

10. Which country consumes the most cheese?
    Greece, followed by France and Italy

11. This dish, which originated in Switzerland, is made from melted cheese into which bread is dipped.
    fondue

12. This pale yellow cheese contains many holes.
    Swiss

13. This hard, dry Italian cheese is usually grated over pasta dishes.
    parmesan

14. People often eat cheese in order to get a sufficient amount of this in their diet. It is especially good for strong bones.
    calcium

15. This mild, very soft cheese, made from curds, is often served with pineapple.
    cottage cheese

16. Wisconsin's Green Bay Packers fans are often called this!
    cheeseheads

FACILITATOR: *This is a great activity to accompany a snack of different types of cheese! Ask participants what their favorite type of cheese is. How much cheese do they eat? Do they like cheese from cows best, or do they prefer goat cheese? Do they like the smell of cheese? Do they think cheese is a healthy snack? Why or why not? Which dishes are the best with cheese?*

Passing Fads

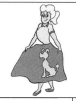

Clothing, decorations, even appliances come and go. What looks so fashionable one year may seem completely silly the next. Take a trip back through fashion time with this worksheet by reading the description and naming the "fad."

1. These pants, popular in the 1970s, were famous for having a wide leg that flared toward the bottom.

2. Popular in the 1950s, these skirts featured a wide swing and an appliqué of an animal or other item on the fabric.

3. These lamps became popular in the 1960s for their colorful glow, which came from heated balls of wax floating in liquid.

4. In the 1980s, these animal figurines became popular as an easy-to-care-for "pet." After applying water and seeds to the pet, a soft, green covering will grow.

5. Many men grew out their hair along the side of their face during the 1960s, making this hairstyle popular.

6. Popular in the 1970s, these "short shorts" were worn tight to emphasize the leg and to create a sexy look.

7. This women's hat was made popular by Jacqueline Kennedy during the 1960s and featured a flat top with straight sides.

8. This "pet" fad was quick to come and go in the 1970s. Many people took part by buying ordinary gray pebbles that came with instructions for care.

9. These outdoor theaters reached the peak of popularity in the 1950s and were a common destination for young lovers and families alike.

10. These large coin-operated music boxes provided plenty of entertainment in restaurants and other establishments and were particularly popular during the 1950s.

11. Originally a sign for victory, it took on a new meaning during the 1960s, when holding the fingers in the shape of a V became popular among war protesters.

12. This type of hat was made from the skin and fur of a raccoon and became especially popular among young boys in the 1950s who were fans of Disney's *Davy Crockett* television show.

13. During the 1960s and '70s, this style of clothing featured bright colors and eclectic patterns and was created by adding dye to fabric.

14. This type of jacket was made popular by the Beatles in the 1960s and is similar to a traditional suit jacket, but has a stand-up collar and fits close to the body.

15. Popular in the 1970s, this suit was a way for men to dress up while also being comfortable.

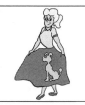

1.   These pants, popular in the 1970s, were famous for having a wide leg that flared toward the bottom.
     bell-bottoms
2.   Popular in the 1950s, these skirts featured a wide swing and an appliqué of an animal or other item on the fabric.
     poodle skirts
3.   These lamps became popular in the 1960s for their colorful glow, which came from heated balls of wax floating in liquid.
     lava lamp
4.   In the 1980s, these animal figurines became popular as an easy-to-care-for "pet." After applying water and seeds to the pet, a soft, green covering will grow.
     Chia Pet
5.   Many men grew out their hair along the side of their face during the 1960s, making this hairstyle popular.
     sideburns
6.   Popular in the 1970s, these "short shorts" were worn tight to emphasize the leg and to create a sexy look.
     hot pants
7.   This women's hat was made popular by Jacqueline Kennedy during the 1960s and featured a flat top with straight sides.
     pillbox hat
8.   This "pet" fad was quick to come and go in the 1970s. Many people took part by buying ordinary gray pebbles that came with instructions for care.
     pet rock
9.   These outdoor theaters reached the peak of popularity in the 1950s and were a common destination for young lovers and families alike.
     drive-in theater
10. These large coin-operated music boxes provided plenty of entertainment in restaurants and other establishments and were particularly popular during the 1950s.
     jukebox
11. Originally a sign for victory, it took on a new meaning during the 1960s, when holding the fingers in the shape of a V became popular among war protesters.
     peace sign
12. This type of hat was made from the skin and fur of a raccoon and became especially popular among young boys in the 1950s who were fans of Disney's *Davy Crockett* television show.
     coonskin hat
13. During the 1960s and '70s, this style of clothing featured bright colors and eclectic patterns and was created by adding dye to fabric.
     tie-dye
14. This type of jacket was made popular by the Beatles in the 1960s and is similar to a traditional suit jacket, but has a stand-up collar and fits close to the body.
     Nehru jacket
15. Popular in the 1970s, this suit was a way for men to dress up while also being comfortable.
     leisure suit

FACILITATOR: *It is likely that many participants wore or collected these items. If you can, bring some of these items into the group for discussion. Some questions to ask: Did you ever own or wear any of these items? What makes something so popular that it becomes a fad? Why are some ideas timeless and others so quick to pass? What are some fads today that will eventually pass?*

Products with Numbers

Products are named in a variety of ways. Manufacturers want a name that will be remembered and will become a "household name." The following products all have a number in their name, such as Bertolli Five Brothers Pasta Sauce. Can you name each product?

1. This steak sauce has been popular for 140 years.

2. This food company, begun in 1892, offered 60 canned and bottled foods at its inception, a few more than its name implies. It has also become a term for a mixed breed of dog.

3. This all-purpose cleaner was first produced by Clorox in 1957.

4. This Campbell's vegetable juice is made from tomatoes and seven other vegetables.

5. This chain of ice-cream parlors has more than 5,600 locations in over 30 countries throughout the world.

6. This lemon-lime soft drink is one of the most popular in the world. It was first launched in 1929 in its original form, but now has additional flavors, such as cherry and mixed berry.

7. This was a popular brand of whiskey and was often mixed with the beverage from the previous question.

8. This is one of the most popular brands of cat food.

9. This petroleum company is famous for its logo, which is an orange ball with numbers written in blue. The company is now owned by ConocoPhillips.

10. This candy bar, made by the Mars Company, is named after "triplets" and has a chocolate and nougat filling.

11. This oil, used as a cleaner, lubricant, and an anti-corrosive solution, is a spray and comes in a familiar bright blue can.

12. This popular vitamin, made by Bayer, is sold separately for men, women, and older adults.

13. This fragrance was first introduced in 1921 and was very popular internationally, especially with women of "high society."

14. This car model, made by Datsun during the 1970s, was a very popular sports car at the time.

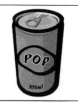

1. This steak sauce has been popular for 140 years.
    A-1

2. This food company, begun in 1892, offered 60 canned and bottled foods at its inception, a few more than its name implies. It has also become a term for a mixed breed of dog.
    Heinz 57

3. This all-purpose cleaner was first produced by Clorox in 1957.
    Formula 409

4. This Campbell's vegetable juice is made from tomatoes and seven other vegetables.
    V8

5. This chain of ice-cream parlors has more than 5,600 locations in over 30 countries throughout the world.
    Baskin-Robbins 31 Ice Cream

6. This lemon-lime soft drink is one of the most popular in the world. It was first launched in 1929 in its original form, but now has additional flavors, such as cherry and mixed berry.
    7UP

7. This was a popular brand of whiskey and was often mixed with the beverage from the previous question.
    Seagram's 7 Crown

8. This is one of the most popular brands of cat food.
    9Lives

9. This petroleum company is famous for its logo, which is an orange ball with numbers written in blue. The company is now owned by ConocoPhillips.
    Union 76

10. This candy bar, made by the Mars Company, is named after "triplets" and has a chocolate and nougat filling.
    3 Musketeers

11. This oil, used as a cleaner, lubricant, and an anti-corrosive solution, is a spray and comes in a familiar bright blue can.
    WD-40

12. This popular vitamin, made by Bayer, is sold separately for men, women, and older adults.
    One A Day

13. This fragrance was first introduced in 1921 and was very popular internationally, especially with women of "high society."
    Chanel No. 5

14. This car model, made by Datsun during the 1970s, was a very popular sports car at the time.
    280Z

FACILITATOR: These products are all well known to most people. What do the participants know about each product? How many have they used? Do they still use them? Are there other similar products that are better? It would add to the activity if you could bring in some of the products or pictures of the products.

Shoes

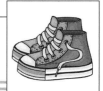

Shoes have evolved from a practical item to protect the feet to a fashion statement that comes in every style and color. Even fictional characters have shown us the importance of a fancy pair of shoes. Through the years shoe fads have fascinated us. Read the description on the left and match it with the answer on the right.

____ 1. Popular in the 1970s, these shoes featured a thick cork sole that added height to the individual wearing them.

a. saddle shoes

____ 2. Frequently worn by children, these shoes have a low heel, closed toe, and a strap with a single buckle across the top.

b. clogs

____ 3. Popular in the 1950s, these two-toned shoes had a white toe and heel and black over the laces and sides.

c. glass slipper

____ 4. These flat athletic shoes were originally introduced in 1916 and were nicknamed "sneakers" because of their rubber sole.

d. Mary Janes

____ 5. In the 1980s, these tennis shoes were popular because of the way they extended to above the ankle.

e. Imelda Marcos

____ 6. This type of shoe is usually a slip-on and has a thick sole that is made of wood.

f. cleats

____ 7. These shoes are made of rubber and are designed to fit over another pair of shoes to protect them from water.

g. platforms

____ 8. These men's dress shoes are generally made of leather and are named for the distinctive "W" pattern on the toe of the shoe.

h. mules

____ 9. Traditionally worn by Native Americans, these soft-soled shoes are made of leather and have fringe or other decorative patterns across the top.

i. Keds

____ 10. These fictional shoes worn by Dorothy in *The Wizard of Oz* were known for their magical powers, which could return Dorothy home anytime she wished.

j. galoshes

____ 11. These shoes are worn in a variety of sports and have studs on the bottom to help a player keep a firm footing.

k. wing tips

____ 12. These boots, popular with women in the 1960s and '70s, had a low heel and were either calf- or knee-high.

l. moccasins

____ 13. This style of shoe is popular with women and has a closed toe and open back and can be low- or high-heeled.

m. penny loafers

____ 14. Known for her collection of over 3,000 shoes, this former first lady of the Philippines is a controversial figure.

n. high tops

____ 15. These laceless shoes were popular in the 1960s, were made of leather, and had an opening to hold a coin.

o. go-go boots

____ 16. In the fairy tale *Cinderella*, this lost shoe led the character to meet and marry the prince.

p. ruby slippers

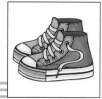

1. Popular in the 1970s, these shoes featured a thick cork sole that added height to the individual wearing them.

    g. platforms

2. Frequently worn by children, these shoes have a low heel, closed toe, and a strap with a single buckle across the top.

    d. Mary Janes

3. Popular in the 1950s, these two-toned shoes had a white toe and heel and black over the laces and sides.

    a. saddle shoes

4. These flat athletic shoes were originally introduced in 1916 and were nicknamed "sneakers" because of their rubber sole.

    i. Keds

5. In the 1980s, these tennis shoes were popular because of the way they extended to above the ankle.

    n. high tops

6. This type of shoe is usually a slip-on and has a thick sole that is made of wood.

    b. clogs

7. These shoes are made of rubber and are designed to fit over another pair of shoes to protect them from water.

    j. galoshes

8. These men's dress shoes are generally made of leather and are named for the distinctive "W" pattern on the toe of the shoe.

    k. wing tips

9. Traditionally worn by Native Americans, these soft-soled shoes are made of leather and have fringe or other decorative patterns across the top.

    l. moccasins

10. These fictional shoes worn by Dorothy in *The Wizard of Oz* were known for their magical powers, which could return Dorothy home anytime she wished.

    p. ruby slippers

11. These shoes are worn in a variety of sports and have studs on the bottom to help a player keep a firm footing.

    f. cleats

12. These boots, popular with women in the 1960s and '70s, had a low heel and were either calf- or knee-high.

    o. go-go boots

13. This style of shoe is popular with women and has a closed toe and open back and can be low- or high-heeled.

    h. mules

14. Known for her collection of over 3,000 shoes, this former first lady of the Philippines is a controversial figure.

    e. Imelda Marcos

15. These laceless shoes were popular in the 1960s, were made of leather, and had an opening to hold a coin.

    m. penny loafers

16. In the fairy tale *Cinderella*, this lost shoe led the character to meet and marry the prince.

    c. glass slipper

FACILITATOR: *If possible, bring in samples or pictures of some of the shoes listed. Which ones have group members worn? What type of shoes are their favorites? How many pairs of shoes does the average person own? What other wardrobe items have come in and out of style? Can the shoes you wear affect your mood?*

Show Me the Money

Money is often said to be the root of all evil. It is, however, a necessity. Money has been in existence for over 2,500 years, and it is a very integral part of the world economy today. The following questions all relate to money in a variety of ways. How many can you answer?

1. Jack Paar and then Phil Baker were the hosts of what television quiz show of the early 1950s that got its start in the 1940s on radio?

2. How much do you get for passing GO on a Monopoly board?

3. Whose picture is on the $1 bill? $5? $10? $20?

4. What are some expressions to describe someone who does not like to spend money?

5. This container, made in the shape of an animal, is often used by children to save coins.

6. A place in New York City where the New York Stock Exchange is located.

7. An expression that means "to give one's opinion."

8. This form of gambling, which dates back to 205 BC, involves drawing a name or number for a prize, often a large sum of money.

9. This magazine, the largest selling in the world, started its famous mail sweepstakes in 1962.

10. This term, which literally means "the cleaning of money," is defined as the transfer of illegally obtained money through a third party to conceal the true source of the money.

11. This is a commonly known list, published annually, of America's wealthiest corporations.

12. There is one main mint in the United States as well as three branches. Where are they each located?

13. This coin, worth a dollar, depicts a woman famous for her work as part of the suffrage movement and was minted only for a short time due to its lack of popularity.

14. Which government bureau prints the United States currency?

15. Give two names that are commonly used as replacements for the word *money*.

16. A name for someone who carries around a lot of money.

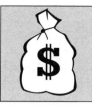

1. Jack Paar and then Phil Baker were the hosts of what television quiz show of the early 1950s that got its start in the 1940s on radio?
   The $64,000 Question

2. How much do you get for passing GO on a Monopoly board?
   $200

3. Whose picture is on the $1 bill? $5? $10? $20?
   Washington, Lincoln, Hamilton, Jackson

4. What are some expressions to describe someone who does not like to spend money?
   frugal, cheap, tightwad, penny-pincher, miser

5. This container, made in the shape of an animal, is often used by children to save coins.
   piggy bank

6. A place in New York City where the New York Stock Exchange is located.
   Wall Street

7. An expression that means "to give one's opinion."
   give one's two-cents' worth

8. This form of gambling, which dates back to 205 BC, involves drawing a name or number for a prize, often a large sum of money.
   lottery

9. This magazine, the largest selling in the world, started its famous mail sweepstakes in 1962.
   Reader's Digest

10. This term, which literally means "the cleaning of money," is defined as the transfer of illegally obtained money through a third party to conceal the true source of the money.
    money laundering

11. This is a commonly known list, published annually, of America's wealthiest corporations.
    Fortune 500

12. There is one main mint in the United States as well as three branches. Where are they each located?
    Denver (CO), Philadelphia (PA), San Francisco (CA), and West Point (NY)

13. This coin, worth a dollar, depicts a woman famous for her work as part of the suffrage movement and was minted only for a short time due to its lack of popularity.
    Susan B. Anthony dollar

14. Which government bureau prints the United States currency?
    Bureau of Printing and Engraving

15. Give two names that are commonly used as replacements for the word *money*.
    dough, moola, greenbacks, bucks, green

16. A name for someone who carries around a lot of money.
    moneybags

FACILITATOR: *Money is always an interesting topic and one that will surely raise many comments. It would be helpful to have U.S. currency and coins as well as money from other countries, if possible, to study and compare. Did participants have a piggy bank when they were young? How do they save money now? Would they consider themselves frugal? Have they ever entered the Reader's Digest sweepstakes or a lottery? Have they owned stocks and bonds? Do they "play" the stock market?*

The Sound of Music

Webster's Dictionary defines music as vocal, instrumental, or mechanical sounds having rhythm, melody, or harmony. For most of us, music is an integral part of our lives, whether by listening, playing, singing, or composing. The following questions relate to music in a variety of ways. How many can you answer?

1. Which stringed instrument is commonly used in bluegrass music?

2. How many types of music can you name?

3. This pluck-stringed, usually triangular-shaped instrument is said to be played by angels floating on clouds. Its strings are perpendicular to the soundboard.

4. This musical instrument, played on a keyboard, is often used for accompaniment. One of the most popular types is the Baby Grand.

5. This boogie-woogie, ragtime style of music is played on the instrument described in question number 4.

6. Many churches have one of these, which consists of sets of pipes.

7. The most popular music lessons taken by children are with this instrument.

8. This classification of musical instruments, often used to accompany, includes the drums, tambourines, bells, cymbals, and congas.

9. This group of four people sings harmoniously without musical accompaniment. The group often wears colorful outfits, bow ties, and boater hats.

10. This stringed instrument in the violin family was first crafted by a famous Italian family in the 1600s and represents a high standard of excellence. Jack Benny often used it in his comedy routine.

11. This Austrian capital is one of the great music cities of the world.

12. This southern U.S. city is often said to be the birthplace of jazz.

13. The Grand Ole Opry in this town is the center of country music.

14. How many string instruments can you name?

The Sound of Music ANSWER SHEET

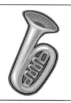

1. Which stringed instrument is commonly used in bluegrass music?
   banjo or mandolin

2. How many types of music can you name?
   opera, folk, rock and roll, country, western, rap, jazz, blues, religious, flamenco, orchestra, marching band, and so forth.

3. This pluck-stringed, usually triangular-shaped instrument is said to be played by angels floating on clouds. Its strings are perpendicular to the soundboard.
   harp

4. This musical instrument, played on a keyboard, is often used for accompaniment. One of the most popular types is the Baby Grand.
   piano

5. This boogie-woogie, ragtime style of music is played on the instrument described in question number 4.
   honky-tonk

6. Many churches have one of these, which consists of sets of pipes.
   organ

7. The most popular music lessons taken by children are with this instrument.
   piano

8. This classification of musical instruments, often used to accompany, includes the drums, tambourines, bells, cymbals, and congas.
   percussion

9. This group of four people sings harmoniously without musical accompaniment. The group often wears colorful outfits, bow ties, and boater hats.
   barbershop quartet

10. This stringed instrument in the violin family was first crafted by a famous Italian family in the 1600s and represents a high standard of excellence. Jack Benny often used it in his comedy routine.
    Stradivarius

11. This Austrian capital is one of the great music cities of the world.
    Vienna

12. This southern U.S. city is often said to be the birthplace of jazz.
    New Orleans

13. The Grand Ole Opry in this town is the center of country music.
    Nashville

14. How many string instruments can you name?
    violin, viola, harp, guitar, cello, bass, harpsichord, lute, mandolin, ukulele, dulcimer, autoharp, and so forth.

FACILITATOR: *This activity would be strengthened if you could bring in some instruments for a "show and tell." Talk about the different types of instruments, places where music is especially popular, types of music, which types participants like best, which instruments they like best, and so forth. Did they ever play an instrument? Do they still? Did they ever make their own "kitchen band" instruments?*

Things that Are Square

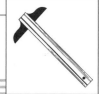

A square is a figure with four equal sides. Not only is *square* used in geometric terms, it also describes a game board, a city block, a dull person, and more. Often the word *square* within an expression means fairness and equality. The following activity deals with a variety of things that are *square*. How many can you name?

1. The following squares are tourist attractions located throughout the world. Can you name the city?

   a. Herald Square in _____

   b. Red Square in _____

   c. Times Square in _____

   d. Tiananmen Square in _____

   e. St. Peter's Square in _____

   f. Trafalgar Square in _____

   g. Union Square in _____

   h. Jackson Square in _____

2. This New York City sports arena is one of the best known in the world and is home to the New York Knicks.

3. This activity is done to music, with four couples facing off against each other to start and then following the instructions of the "caller."

4. In mathematical terms, the _____ of 9 is 3, because 3 × 3 = 9.

5. This technical instrument is used to draw perpendicular lines.

6. This ball game is played among players on a square court divided into four equal parts. It is enjoyed on playgrounds around the United States.

7. This is the area in the center of many small cities.

8. The follow descriptions are of common phrases that contain the word *square*:

   a. A nourishing and substantial meal. _____

   b. To have to go back and start over. _____

   c. To be honest and straightforward. _____

   d. To eat three nutritious meals a day. _____

   e. When one is in a place where he or she just doesn't fit in and feels out of place. _____

   f. When one takes a stance to begin a fight. _____

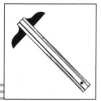

Things that Are Square ANSWER SHEET

1. The following squares are tourist attractions located throughout the world. Can you name the city?
   a. **Herald Square (New York City)**
   b. **Red Square (Moscow)**
   c. **Times Square (New York City)**
   d. **Tiananmen Square (Beijing)**
   e. **St. Peter's Square (Rome)**
   f. **Trafalgar Square (London)**
   g. **Union Square (San Francisco)**
   h. **Jackson Square (New Orleans)**

2. This New York City sports arena is one of the best known in the world and is home to the New York Knicks.
   Madison Square Garden

3. This activity is done to music, with four couples facing off against each other to start and then following the instructions of the "caller."
   square dance

4. In mathematical terms, the _____ of 9 is 3, because $3 \times 3 = 9$.
   square root

5. This ruler is used to draw perpendicular lines.
   T square

6. This ball game is played among players on a square court divided into four equal parts. It is enjoyed on playgrounds around the United States.
   four squares

7. This is the area in the center of many small cities.
   town square

8. The follow descriptions are of common phrases that contain the word *square*. Can you name the phrase?
   a. **A nourishing and substantial meal.**   square meal
   b. **To have to go back and start over.**   back to square one
   c. **To be honest and straightforward.**   fair and square
   d. **To eat three nutritious meals a day.**   eat three squares a day
   e. **When one is in a place where he or she just doesn't fit in and feels out of place.**   square peg in a round hole
   f. **When one takes a stance to begin a fight.**   square off

FACILITATOR: This activity is broad based so that conversations can go in a number of different directions. How many participants have been to any of the famous squares? Has anyone ever been square dancing? Do they know of any other expressions that use the word square? Looking around, how many things can participants name that are square? Depending on the group, you might want to ask for the square roots of a few numbers, too.

Strengthen Your Mind, Volume Two by Einberger & Sellick. Copyright © 2008 by Health Professions Press, Inc.

Things with a Letter in Their Name

There are many items used in everyday life that have a letter in their name. Some letters are used as abbreviations, while others are just part of the name of the item. For this worksheet, read the description and write the answer in the space provided. Each answer will have a single letter as part of the name of the item.

1. This bomber plane is used by the United States Air Force and is sometimes called "The Bone."

2. A police dog team is sometimes referred to as a _____ unit.

3. This mountain in the Himalayas is the second highest mountain on Earth.

4. This type of assault rifle is commonly used in the United States military.

5. In the medical field, this type of picture is commonly used to see bones or other internal body structures.

6. Major Hollywood movie stars who command millions of dollars per film are sometimes referred to as this.

7. This rating is given to films that are appropriate for even the youngest children.

8. This sport is often played by children as an introduction to baseball.

9. This popular candy is known by the slogan "Melts in your mouth, not in your hands."

10. In science, this is used to measure the acceleration of an object.

11. When someone tries hard, it is said that he or she earns an _____ for effort.

12. This popular corn and wheat cereal is made by Kellogg's.

13. This device is used for cleaning wax out of the ears.

14. On this popular Web site individuals can "bid" on and purchase items.

15. This popular discount store is known for its blue-light specials.

1. This bomber plane is used by the United States Air Force and is sometimes called "The Bone."
   B-2

2. A police dog team is sometimes referred to as a _____ unit.
   K-9

3. This mountain in the Himalayas is the second highest mountain on Earth.
   K2

4. This type of assault rifle is commonly used in the United States military.
   M-16

5. In the medical field, this type of picture is commonly used to see bones or other internal body structures.
   x-ray

6. Major Hollywood movie stars who command millions of dollars per film are sometimes referred to as this.
   A-list

7. This rating is given to films that are appropriate for even the youngest children.
   G

8. This sport is often played by children as an introduction to baseball.
   T-ball

9. This popular candy is known by the slogan "Melts in your mouth, not in your hands."
   M&M's

10. In science, this is used to measure the acceleration of an object.
    G-force

11. When someone tries hard, it is said that he or she earns an _____ for effort.
    A

12. This popular corn and wheat cereal is made by Kellogg's.
    Special K

13. This device is used for cleaning wax out of the ears.
    Q-tip

14. On this popular Web site individuals can "bid" on and purchase items.
    eBay

15. This popular discount store is known for its blue-light specials.
    Kmart

FACILITATOR: *Discussion of letters can go in so many different directions. How did these items get their name? Is the letter in the name short for another word? In movies, what other ratings are used other than the G rating? What are some other letter abbreviations that are used in the military? Are there other items used in everyday life that have letter abbreviations? Bring in some M&M's for the group to enjoy. For an extra mental workout, try an A–Z list of abbreviations.*

What's What in American Business?

There are hundreds of thousands of businesses in the United States, from small home-based businesses to giant multi-billion-dollar corporations that employ thousands of people. Those that we know best, outside of our own community, are usually those that are among the largest in their field. The following facts all relate to one of the giants in a particular industry. How many businesses can you name?

1. This large department store has hosted a Thanksgiving Day parade in New York City for nearly 100 years.

2. This store, started by Sam Walton, is one of the largest corporations in the world.

3. This fast-food restaurant with golden arches, the largest in the world, was established in 1940 and is now located in 120 countries worldwide.

4. This was one of the first five-and-dime stores in the United States and was well known for its luncheon counters.

5. This business, established in 1888, is the largest information technology employer and overall most profitable computer company in the world.

6. This large oil company is perhaps most famous for the Valdez oil spill in Alaska in 1989, which killed hundreds of thousands of animals of various types.

7. This international department store, established in the United States in the late 1800s, was especially well known in its early years for its famous catalog.

8. This is the largest bank in the United States.

9. This is the leading manufacturer of farming equipment in the world.

10. This company, one of the largest in radio, took over the Victor Talking Machine Company in 1929.

11. This is the largest greeting card company in the United States, accounting for over half of all cards sent each year.

12. This company, started in 1916 by a man of the same name, is one of the world's largest producers of aircraft.

13. Bill Gates is the head of this American multinational computer technology corporation, one of the largest in the world.

14. This corporation, based in Detroit, Michigan, is the largest automobile producer in the world.

15. This U.S. toy company, established in 1945 and one of the world's largest, manufactures some of the most well-known toys, including Barbie dolls.

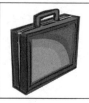

1. This large department store has hosted a Thanksgiving Day parade in New York City for nearly 100 years.
   Macy's
2. This store, started by Sam Walton, is one of the largest corporations in the world.
   Wal-Mart
3. This fast-food restaurant with golden arches, the largest in the world, was established in 1940 and is now located in 120 countries worldwide.
   McDonald's
4. This was one of the first five-and-dime stores in the United States and was well known for its luncheon counters.
   Woolworth's
5. This business, established in 1888, is the largest information technology employer and overall most profitable computer company in the world.
   IBM
6. This large oil company is perhaps most famous for the Valdez oil spill in Alaska in 1989, which killed hundreds of thousands of animals of various types.
   Exxon
7. This international department store, established in the United States in the late 1800s, was especially well known in its early years for its famous catalog.
   Sears Roebuck
8. This is the largest bank in the United States.
   Bank of America
9. This is the leading manufacturer of farming equipment in the world.
   John Deere (Deere & Company)
10. This company, one of the largest in radio, took over the Victor Talking Machine Company in 1929.
    RCA
11. This is the largest greeting card company in the United States, accounting for over half of all cards sent each year.
    Hallmark
12. This company, started in 1916 by a man of the same name, is one of the world's largest producers of aircraft.
    Boeing
13. Bill Gates is the head of this American multinational computer technology corporation, one of the largest in the world.
    Microsoft
14. This corporation, based in Detroit, Michigan, is the largest automobile producer in the world.
    General Motors
15. This U.S. toy company, established in 1945 and one of the world's largest, manufactures some of the most well-known toys, including Barbie dolls.
    Mattel

FACILITATOR: We often have a fascination with large companies. Some people prefer to shop at the largest stores or buy from the largest manufacturers. Others prefer to shop at small, locally owned stores and buy from smaller manufacturers. Which do participants prefer? What do they think of these companies? Have they shopped at these places or bought these brands? How do they rate these businesses? Did they buy gas from Exxon after the oil spill? Did they eat at Woolworth's luncheon counters? Have they watched the Macy's Thanksgiving Day parade? Have they owned a General Motors car? Have they eaten a McDonald's hamburger?

Where on the Human Body?

The human body is amazing, as it goes about many of its functions without us even knowing. It has the power to heal itself when injured and to create new life. In this worksheet, you will take a tour of the fabulous body.

1. How many bones does the human body have?
   a. 90
   b. 156
   c. 206

2. How much blood is in the human body?
   a. 3 pints
   b. 10 pints
   c. 15 pints

3. What is the largest organ in the body?

4. There are several organs that, if removed, one can live without. How many can you name?

5. Of all the bones in the body, which one is the easiest to break?

6. The rib cage, ear, and nose are all home to this type of tissue.

7. What part of the body is considered the least sensitive?

8. Technology has made it possible to improve parts of the body that do not work as well as they should. Name at least three of these corrective devices.

9. An artificial limb designed to function as a real body part is called a what?

10. How long does it take blood to circulate once around the body?
    a. 60 seconds
    b. 3 minutes
    c. 5 minutes

11. Other than the fingerprint, what "print" is unique to each individual person?

12. Of all the types of hair on the body, which grows the fastest?
    a. arm
    b. beard
    c. head

13. Where on the body would you find the following?
    a. tibia _____
    b. Achilles tendon _____
    c. mandible _____
    d. femur _____
    e. bicep _____
    f. jugular _____
    g. ulna _____
    h. pinna _____
    i. coccyx _____
    j. rotator cuff _____
    k. patella _____

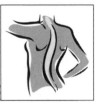

1. How many bones does the human body have?
    c. **206**

2. How much blood is in the human body?
    b. **10 pints**

3. What is the largest organ in the body?
    skin

4. There are several organs that, if removed, one can live without. How many can you name?
    gall bladder, pancreas, appendix, one kidney, one lung

5. Of all the bones in the body, which one is the easiest to break?
    clavicle (or collar bone)

6. The rib cage, ear, and nose are all home to this type of tissue.
    cartilage

7. What part of the body is considered the least sensitive?
    middle of back or shoulder

8. Technology has made it possible to improve parts of the body that do not work as well as they should. Name at least three of these corrective devices.
    hearing aid, eyeglasses, braces, dentures, pacemaker

9. An artificial limb designed to function as a real body part is called a what?
    prosthesis

10. How long does it take blood to circulate once around the body?
    a. **60 seconds**

11. Other than the fingerprint, what "print" is unique to each individual person?
    tongue print

12. Of all the types of hair on the body, which grows the fastest?
    b. **beard**

13. Where on the body would you find the following?
    a. **tibia: large bone in the lower leg**
    b. **Achilles tendon: above the heel**
    c. **mandible: jawbone**
    d. **femur: thighbone**
    e. **bicep: muscle on the front of the upper arm**
    f. **jugular: vein on either side of the neck**
    g. **ulna: smaller bone of the lower arm**
    h. **pinna: outer ear**
    i. **coccyx: tailbone**
    j. **rotator cuff: shoulder joint**
    k. **patella: knee cap**

FACILITATOR: *Bring in a "map" of the human body for participants to refer to when discussing the worksheet. Encourage discussion by asking the following questions: Have you ever had an organ removed? Have you ever broken a bone? Which one? What medical advances are readily available today as compared to 50 years ago? Plastic surgery is used regularly to improve people's looks. Would you ever consider it?*